CHILD DEVELOPMENT

CHILD DEVELOPMENT

(In 3 Volumes)

Health and Nutrition for the School-age Child

(Volume-2)

Dr. Sujata Mittal

ISHA BOOKS
DELHI-110 033

Child Development

Rs. 2500 (Set)
Rs. 835 (each volume)

ISBN: 81-8205-085-5 (Set)
ISBN: 81-8205-087-1 (Vol. 2)

Published in 2004 in India by
Isha Books, D-43, Prithviraj Road,
Adarsh Nagar, Delhi-110 033

Laser Typesetting at : Shree Vaishnavi Creations, Delhi
Printed at : Chawla Offset Press, Delhi

Contents

Preface

Children of school age face health and nutrition problems that may affect their individual physical development, their capacity to attend school and their ability to learn. The aetiology of impaired cognitive development is now a central area for concern while improvements in cognitive performance produce opportunities for evaluating the impact of school health and nutrition programmes.

The main nutritional problems faced by the school-age child include stunting, underweight, anaemia, deficiency of iodine and deficiency of vitamin A. In countries experiencing the nutrition transition, overweight and obesity are growing problems in the school-age child. Other common health problems faced by children of this age-group include helminth infections, malaria, diarrhoeal diseases, respiratory infections and tuberculosis. Much of the disease burden derives from bad diet, poor environmental conditions and a lack of resources essential for human health.

Good nutrition is the base of good health. However, most people are ignorant of the proper ways and means to maintain good health and nutrition. Food taboos and antiquated food beliefs and practices that have been passed on for generations have always been a great barrier to modifying eating behaviours or habits. Functional illiteracy related to malnutrition and the poor learning environment in rural settings and among disadvantaged urban groups are among the ecological factors that maintain the vicious cycle leading to malnutrition. In order to break this cycle, an effective means of continuously transferring information on sound nutrition is imperative.

The present volume offers a comprehensive review of the latest information on nutrition, physical activity, eating disorders, and prevention of chronic disease in childhood. It identifies important health considerations for child, describes previous interventions and current behaviour patterns, identifies gaps in current knowledge, and recommends ways to improve nutrition and fitness in children and adolescents. It will serve as a valuable reference tool for medical and nutrition professionals, school and public health personnel, physical educators, and others involved in promoting child health.

Editor

1

School Health and Nutrition Analysis

The health problems that begin in childhood and adolescence but that manifest themselves later in life - HIV infection, for example, and tobacco use. Besides the causes of disease and death, information should ideally include the age and sex of subjects, their location and its geography (e.g. whether urban or rural, wet or dry) and the season during which they became ill. Interventions designed subsequent to the situation analysis can then be carefully targeted.

The primary causes of absenteeism may not be among the major health issues, but identifying ways to reduce absenteeism is critical if children are to receive schooling and school-based health and nutrition interventions. Information on the extent of the non-formal education sector may reveal further opportunities to deliver nutrition and health education and services.

The non-formal sector may be important for particular groups such as girls or adolescents that may be underserved by the formal sector. Information should cover laws on sexual harassment by teachers, laws restricting access to tobacco and alcohol, policies on sex education, and policies on allowing school-age girls who become pregnant to return to school.

Current community spending on the education, nutrition and health of school-age children. This information will indicate the potential for school nutrition and health programmes to achieve sustainability through community contributions and other community approaches to cost recovery.

Of interest are not only existing school programmes but also the general health services intended for school-age children. Information on the availability of material and financial resources will be particularly important in assessing local resource capacity and response. Basic topics include:

— *The specific responsibilities of the health and education sectors for school nutrition and health education and services;*

— *National and regional policies relating to school nutrition and health programmes - their relevance and the extent to which they are open for review;*

— *The structure, components, and coverage of any existing school nutrition and health programmes, including customary health screening and first aid programmes;*

— *Current approaches to health education, including family life and reproductive health education, and other nutrition- and health-related activities such as school health clubs;*

- *Current use of primary health care facilities by the school-age group, including use of reproductive health facilities, and referrals between schools and the primary health care system;*
- *The extent to which school-age children use private health services and traditional healers;*
- *The content, coverage, effectiveness and cost of school feeding programmes and school gardens;*
- *Information on school canteens and local food vendors who serve schools;*
- *Information on school water supply and sanitary and waste disposal facilities;*
- *The contribution of NGOs and intergovernmental organisations to school programmes;*
- *The community's contribution to schools and health including the provision of clean water and good sanitation facilities, school feeding, and other nutrition and health services;*
- *Current levels of investment by government or other agencies in the health and nutrition of school-age children;*
- *Pre-school and special education provision.*

UNICEF situation analyses of the education and health sectors might contain information on some of these items or may provide a basis for comparison. For example, one informative comparison would be that between the quality of water and sanitation in the school and the quality of water and sanitation in the household and the community.

These resources will come from the many sectors relevant to health and education (governmental, non-governmental, and intergovernmental) and even from the children themselves and the wider community. Information is also necessary on the financial and economic cost of proposed interventions. These entities include sports and religious organisations, social welfare groups and the media. Contributions from such sources may be particularly important in ensuring sustainability of school health and nutrition programmes.

School Health and Nutrition Programmes

There have been substantial reductions in child death rates, gains in health, immunization levels, improved nutrition programmes and disease prevention over the last 50 years. UNICEF estimates that more than 90% of the world's children are now surviving beyond the age of 5 years. As a result there are now more children of school age and a higher proportion of children attending school than ever before.

Despite the improvements in survival of school-aged children, there is still a major burden of disease and ill health among this group, particularly in areas such as poor nutrition and intestinal parasitic diseases. This burden of ill health compromises the children's development, school attendance and ability to take advantage of what may be their only opportunity to obtain a formal education. Improving the health and learning of school children through school-based health and nutrition programmes is not a new concept.

Many countries have school health programmes, and many agencies have decades of experience. These common experiences suggest an opportunity for concerted action by a partnership of agencies to broaden the scope of school health programmes and make them more effective. An interagency initiative, that includes WHO, UNICEF, UNESCO and the World Bank, has identified a core group of activities, each already recommended by the participating agencies, that captures the best practices from programme experiences.

This core group of activities consists of health-related school policies; provision of safe water and sanitation; skills based health education and school based health and nutrition services. Focusing initially on these activities will allow concerted action by the participating agencies, and will ensure consistent advice to country programmes and projects. Because of the simplicity of this approach, it will increase the number of countries able to implement school health components of child-friendly school reforms, and help ensure that these programmes go to scale.

The focused actions are seen as a starting point to which other interventions may be added, as appropriate. The current survey of donor and agency support of school based health and nutrition programmes aims to give an overview of major areas of donor support, policies and interests. It also serves to highlight areas that are still of great concern. These include the problems of HIV/AIDS infection and that of girls' access to education.

World Health Organisation (WHO)

The World Health Organization is the UN agency that

is the coordinating authority for international health work. In 1996, WHO launched the Global School Health Initiative (GSHI) which aims to increase the number of schools that can be called "health promoting" schools (HPS). A HPS is defined as a school that "constantly strengthens its capacity as a healthy setting for living, learning and working".

Within WHO this initiative is coordinated by a multi-sectoral working group that incorporates expertise in mental health and Life Skills Training (LST), health and nutrition, physical environments etc. Some 22 WHO divisions are relevant to school health strategy, and 8 of these are represented in a coordinating group. WHO also collaborates with other UN organisations and with the World Bank. WHO is a cosponsor of PCD.

Four broad strategies have been identified to help schools become health promoting:

- *Building capacity to advocate for improved school health programmes*
- *Mobilising resources for developing Health Promoting Schools*
- *Strengthening national capacities*
- *Research to improve school health programmes*

This initiative emphasises the need to harness existing resources that exist at country, community and school level whilst also assisting governments to advocate for increased funds for HPS. The focus therefore is on influencing government policy through advocacy and the longer term sustainability of the initiative. To date, a broad range of advocacy orientated activities have been implemented under the auspices of WHO.

This includes the development of guidelines and action plans by task force members, training and workshop based activities and the production of key documents that provide an important entry point for the development of Health Promoting Schools. Documents have been produced that address important technical issues such as: the reduction of helminth infections; the prevention of violence; HIV/AIDS/STD prevention; the dangers of tobacco use and the improvement of nutritional status. These documents are intended for use by governments and those concerned with advocating the allocation of greater resources for school health.

Although all seven WHO regional offices are actively involved in supporting this initiative, they are at various stages of development and employ different entry points to HPS depending on the regional location. In Fujian, China, for example, WHO have been supporting a project for de-worming since 1996 as an entry point to the development of HPS. A pilot study was undertaken to demonstrate the benefits of de-worming and health education.

In addition, the HPS project has become a trigger for activities that improved the physical environment through mobilising local government and community funds. These improvements included tree planting, extending the school buildings, increased numbers of toilets and taps for handwashing and other general environmental improvements. WHO has also supported research on school based health services through the Task Force for Healthy School Children, within WHO/ Special Programme for Research and Training in Tropical Diseases (TDR).

This Task Force, within which PCD was represented, undertook enabling research on school based health service delivery, and field tested the UNICEF-led inter-agency Situation Analysis in Africa. The Division of Control of Tropical Disease (CTD) has conducted school based deworming activities in Zanzibar, Seychelles, Oman and Mauritius and has worked with World Bank projects in West Africa to design school based health service delivery of anthelmintics.

The Division is currently establishing a formal collaboration with the World Bank to support school based deworming projects. WHO has set a target of 75% coverage with regular anthelmintic treatment of school-age children in countries where helminth infections are a public health problem. The Pan American Health Organisation has a well established network of health promoting schools in the Americas. Schools are also the basis of health delivery for the 'PEPIN' disease control initiative that is active in Nicaragua, El Salvador, Guatemala and Honduras, and is currently expanding to 12 other countries. In October 1997, the World Bank and PAHO launched a joint initiative to promote school health and nutrition programmes in the Americas.

Pan American Health Organistion (PAHO)

PAHO is an international public health agency with more than 90 years of experience in working to improve the health and living standards of the countries of the Americas. It serves as the specialised organization for health of the Inter-American System. It also serves as the Regional Office for the Americas of the World Health Organization. PAHO works in all the countries of the region of the Americas, including the Caribbean. They have offices (called Representations) in 29 countries, each with a health promotion consultant who works directly with the Ministry of health and Education, as well as NGOs and teacher training colleges to strengthen school health programmes in the context of the Health Promoting Schools Initiative (HPSI).

PAHO's policy towards the school-age child is to promote the development of life skills, in the context of the HPSI, as well as to provide early detection, preventing services and primary health care through the schools and the health service structure in each country. The HPSI is a school based health promotion strategy, supporting through technical cooperation.

Most of PAHO's work is in advocacy to strengthen school policies and programs that go beyond traditional screening and school feeding programs, to integrate health promotion activities, especially life skills and to establish risk factor surveillance (behaviours and conditions) as a school based research activity. The HPSI strategy includes the following components:

— *Needs assessment to identify strengths and weaknesses in school health programs.*

— *Review of policy and programs, with establishment or strengthening of joint commissions to coordinate school health activities between Health and Education sectors.*

— *Review and up-date of school health curriculum.*

— *Review and up-date of teacher training programs.*

— *Establishment of life skills education.*

— *Establishment of youth risk behaviour surveillance.*

— *Evaluation of health promoting capacity of schools.*

Based on the results of a needs assessment, the HPSI integrates health requirements and interventions into a comprehensive strategy. Other programs in PAHO deal with specific issues, such as HIV/AIDS, helminth infection (Division of Disease Prevention and Control), nutrition education guidelines and micronutrient supplementation (Food and Nutrition Program), water and sanitation (Health and Environment Division).

PAHO and the World Bank established a Partnership to support school health programs in 1997, and in the context of this partnership have prepared joint documents and are in the process of preparing a joint publication on the school health situation in LAC, including case studies to highlight some good practices in depth.

Food and Agricultural Organisation (FAO)

FAO's approach towards the health of school aged children is guided by the resolutions approved at the International Conference on Nutrition in December 1992 and further reconfirmed at the World Food Summit in 1996. FAO's current focus is on consolidating and expanding a programme on Nutrition Education in Primary Schools (NEPS), initiated in collaboration with the Netherlands Nutrition Center.

This programme evolved from a survey in 55

countries Worldwide, which revealed the need for nutrition-related materials in primary schools and for teacher training in the use of these materials. The NEPS programme of FAO aims at promoting interest in school-based nutrition education and assisting developing countries in the planning of such activities in primary schools.

The curriculum for a preparatory course for professionals, who will become facilitators of the planning process with teachers, has also been developed and will be tested in the first quarter of 2000. The next step is to utilise these materials to assist countries in developing their own nutrition education programmes and to prepare teaching and learning materials on nutrition for children between the ages of six and fourteen. These materials will have to be appropriate to the local food and nutrition situation and to the level of detail and institutional capacity of the country of concern.

For example, some countries may wish to incorporate nutrition education into the education curriculum while others will want to use the materials in a less structured way. By simultaneously addressing pupils, teachers, school personnel, parents and the community - an approach the NEPS programme is emphasising - it is possible to accelerate improvement in both the learning and living environments of the students. FAO's strategy on nutrition education in schools fits well within the concept of health promoting schools as defined by World Health Organization (WHO). Accordingly, FAO is actively collaborating in the world-wide School Health Initiative, promoted by the WHO and its respective regional networks for health promoting schools.

World Food Programme (WFP)

WFP is concerned with two main areas in relation to school health: school feeding programmes and a micronutrient and health programme. These form part of the WFP's 'Food-for-Growth' objectives, with projects that target needy people at the most critical times of their lives: babies, school children, pregnant and breast feeding women and the elderly. WFP has a long-standing role in support of School Feeding Programmes (SFP) and supports around 60 programmes today.

SFPs are increasingly targeted at poor countries and poor population groups within these countries: by the end of 1997 90% of WFP resources were to be directed at low-income food deficit countries. SFPs are justified on the basis that they contribute to improvements in school enrolment and attendance rates, improvements in children's capacity to concentrate and assimilate information by alleviating short-term hunger and because they reduce the prevalence of some micronutrient deficiencies through the provision of fortified foods (Vitamin A, iron and iodine).

Increasingly, school-based de-worming programmes (which follow the WHO technical guidelines) are being integrated into SFPs. Training of ministerial government staff, teachers and health staff at the peripheral level enables them to take responsibility for drug distribution. WFP, in collaboration with WHO, has completed the production of a "Health and Nutrition Manual for School Feeding Programmes".

WFP is also coordinating the Women's Health and Nutrition Facility (WHNF), a programme funded by CIDA. WHNF started in 1996 and is targeted at 15 low-income countries reaching over 900,000 women and 2.2 million children, including the school-aged child. Fortified foods, and specific micronutrients along with de-worming tablets are targeted to the most vulnerable in the population and at the most vulnerable stages in their life. For example, vitamin A is targeted at women during pregnancy.

The programme, costing $30 million (Canadian dollars) is implemented over a 3-4 year period depending on the particular circumstances of the countries involved. Where possible, WFP aims to integrate the programme into their existing regular programmes for example Maternal and Child Health (MCH) and SFP and to work closely with other organisations (e.g. UNICEF) in the target countries.

As one of five key activity areas WFP focuses on projects that promote trade-offs in favour of education for girls and women. When supply of food is short and household income is low, girls' education often suffers, with a decrease in school attendance. Along with 'traditional' school feeding programmes, WFP advocates the wider use of an approach tested in Malawi, Morocco, Niger, Pakistan and Yemen, which involves provision of a ration of food to the family when the daughter attends school, rather than assisting by feeding the child at school.

In its food aid programmes WFP works with various partners within the framework of national policy. Partners may include local governments and national Ministries along with national and internal

NGOs and other UN agencies such as WHO, UNICEF, UNESCO and FAO.

United Nations Children's Fund (UNICEF)

UNICEF's medium-term strategy for 1996-2001 has identified women and young people as two main priority groups. Their policy is to help meet the basic rights and expand opportunities of children aged 0 to 18 within the framework of the 1989 UN Convention of the Rights of the Child, the 1990 World Summit for Children and the 1990 World Conference "Education for All" (EFA).

In addition, UNICEF's mandate is to support WHO and UNESCO policies and develop common strategies that address school health and the joint UN Programme on AIDS, which improves coverage and quality of school-based life skills/AIDS programmes. They also work within the Framework for Girls Education (1996) and take guidance from the Notebook on Programming for Young People's Health and Development.

UNICEF's Programme Priorities for 1998-2000 target key World Summit for Children goals, such as increased immunization coverage and improved access to education, in countries where progress is most needed. UNICEF is also part of the joint WHO Roll Back Malaria Campaign. UNICEF has been involved with school health programmes for many years and collaborates with a number of agencies including the World Bank, WHO, UNESCO and UNFPA.

Recently UNICEF has worked in some depth with several countries (Cameroon, Eastern Caribbean, Ghana,

Sri Lanka, Thailand and Zimbabwe) on school health programme policy. Currently UNICEF supports a range of school health programmes in the following areas:

- *Water, Sanitation and Hygiene programmes for schools in many countries. These include health education courses in primary schools that focus on hygiene and the environment, provision of facilities for safe water, latrines, handwashing and garbage disposal.*
- *Life skills/AIDS programmes in schools including curriculum training.*
- *Child-to-Child and extra-curricular activities for the whole community, with NGOs, for example: World Scout Federation, Red Cross and Red Cross Crescent Societies.*
- *Health and Nutrition services including the provision of micronutrients, anthelminthics and malaria tablets as part of UNICEF's overall strategy.*
- *Situation Analysis including adolescents' needs and responses. This was developed as an inter-agency (UNDP, UNESCO, UNFPA, WHO) activity, with PCD, and has been evaluated (by WHO) in Ghana, Zimbabwe, Botswana, Uganda and Kenya.*

UNICEF is also currently developing ideas for a package of school based interventions that have the scope for sustainable national adaptation. Currently this package has four components as follows:

- *School Policies: the focus will be country specific but should include protecting children against physical/ sexual abuse, protecting the rights of pregnant schoolgirls, protecting the rights of children who are disabled or are living with HIV/AIDS, and avoiding tobacco and substance abuse.*

— *Skills-based health education/Life Skills Training:* ensuring school children get the skills as well as the information they need (for everything from preventing HIV/AIDS to contributing to civil society), in a way that fosters an interactive relationship between teachers and school children.

— *Water, Sanitation and Hygiene Promotion:* which should be linked to environmental issues and the hygiene component of health education. Schools could possibly act as a central point for community managed water programmes.

— *Specific medical/nutrition interventions:* there are a number of interventions that can be safely and simply implemented by teachers including the regular treatment of helminth infections, micronutrient supplementation (iron, vitamin A and iodine) and possibly, in selected areas, malaria treatment and tetracycline for the treatment of trachoma.

Four programme principles have been identified to support these four interventions:

— *Strengthening partnerships/linkages:* between schools and communities/ parents, between education and the health sector including water and environmental health and between teachers and health workers.

— *Capacity building:* supporting the work teachers are already doing rather than overwhelming them; this includes the provision of training and the production of materials.

— *Sustainability:* seeking long term programmes,

although not necessarily independent of external support.

— *Children's participation: programmes which respond to needs recognised by the beneficiaries, and involving them actively in implementation.*

Many UNICEF country programmes are already supporting elements of the package outlined above. For example in Punjab Province, Pakistan, UNICEF supports the Government Education Department in an integrated water, sanitation and hygiene education project in primary schools (IWSHEP).

The IWSHEP aims to increase access to water and sanitation facilities (through the provision of hand pumps and construction of latrines) in primary schools for girls; to promote hygiene practices and improved health among school-aged children and to strengthen the capacity of the Education Department by improving in-service teacher training which includes a hygiene-education component.

Additional support is targeted at NGO elementary schools to promote personal hygiene awareness and environmental sanitation among primary school children. School children and teachers provide an effective channel for education and appropriate training materials have been developed. About 8000 teachers were trained under the project in 1994.

In Zimbabwe, UNICEF supports a LST/AIDS programme that is now under the Ministry of Education. In 1992 UNICEF gave US$350,000 for the hire of local staff and programme start-up after which a fundraising campaign with local donors led to the raising of US$4 million of supplementary funding for 2 *years. The programme supports weekly (compulsory) lessons on life skills and HIV/AIDS in all schools for children from grade 4 (9-10 years of age).*

Teacher and student manuals are provided which are appropriate for the grade level, which address relationships, growing-up, life skills and health. Self-esteem and assertion are positively encouraged and concrete ways of responding to negative peer pressure are role-played at school. Children undertake community-based projects that explore drug use, coping with HIV/AIDS and responsibilities of husbands and wives.

Whilst many UNICEF country programmes are supporting school health initiatives, these have not yet been adequately tried and tested in order to be formalised within the organisation. It is anticipated that a select number of countries will be identified to pilot the package outlined above and explore the various programming implications before UNICEF formerly adopts the approach as a broad-based strategy.

A body of people with expertise in key areas such as LST, water and sanitation (including hygiene promotion), helminth infection control, interactive health education (including HIV/AIDS) along with representatives of donors and key organisations could be brought together to co-ordinate and catalyse the process. In addition to school based programmes, UNICEF are also considering the more difficult area of reaching children in crises, as well as street children and working children, who are often not attending schools and whose health and nutrition are often most compromised.

United Nations Educational, Scientific and Cultural Organisation (UNESCO)

Promoting safe and supportive environments for development of teaching and learning is an integral part of UNESCO's action. This includes assistance, for example, in providing comfortable and functional classrooms, adequate sanitary conditions at schools, a broad and balanced curriculum or caring interactions between and amongst staff and pupils. Several programmes and projects of UNESCO concern the teaching and learning of health. Health and nutrition education is promoted in collaboration notably with WHO within the framework of the global school health initiative; however, co-operation with other relevant agencies such as UNICEF, World Bank or FAO is also being fostered.

Current activities include national and sub-regional health education projects, teacher training and material development. Health education issues are also mainstreamed throughout the education system, notably within the context of science and technology education, based as they are on similar aims and pedagogical principles providing knowledge and skills to improve the present and future well-being of all.

UNESCO is also fostering the integration of specific health issues such as HIV/AIDS education, prevention of drug abuse, population education and reproductive health in numerous programmes world-wide in collaboration with UNAIDS, UNDCP, UNFPA, Education International and others. In the field of school health services, UNESCO provides technical support for WFP School Feeding Programmes. This includes assistance with the appraisal of new programmes, management reviews, the evaluation of existing SFPs and the development of manuals on different aspects of design and implementation of SFPs.

United Nations Drug Control Programme (UNDCP)

UNDCP works in collaboration with other UN (and non-UN) agencies and organisations to support a number of programmes aimed at drug abuse prevention in young people. An example of UNDCP support is the project 'Young People in Crisis', implemented by UNICEF, UNDCP and other UN agencies, intergovernmental and non-governmental organisations.

The project aims at meeting the health and developmental need of young people, focusing on prevention and reduction of the abuse of drugs, within the context of a comprehensive approach to the health and development of young people. UNDCP supported projects include those aimed at both in-school and out-of-school young people.

Practices used in the projects include peer counselling and education, employed in preventive education and awareness campaigns, as well as the use of alternative activities such as theatre, performance arts and sport. The Global Youth Network project was formed at the "For you, by youth" Global Forum on Drug Abuse Prevention, held at Banff, Alberta, Canada in 1998. The Global Youth Network programmes function as antennas for monitoring emerging trends and as sites for pilot testing of new prevention approaches.

Examples of programmes supported by UNDCP include:

— *The UNDCP/WHO Global Initiative on Primary Prevention of Substance Abuse works through encouragement of healthy lifestyles, equipping youth with tools to cope with stress, peer pressure and other risk factors in substance abuse. Under this initiative, projects will be implemented in central and eastern Europe, southern Africa and south-east Asia. All the projects place strong emphasis on national capacity-building and support and empowerment of local communities.*

— *Joint project with UNICEF in Kenya, integrating drug abuse prevention education into alternative basic education programmes for out-of -school children in Kenya. Activities include the design and implementation of a drug prevention education curriculum and the training of 30 teachers as district teacher trainers who will, in turn, train all other 16 districts.*

— *In Bolivia UNDCP worked with UNICEF in the development and implementation of a night school curriculum for working and street children. This project was intended to develop and implement a new curriculum for the formal education night school programme, with emphasis on a drug abuse prevention component, and to train teachers in the use of the new curriculum and about the special needs of working and street children.*

United Nations Development Programme (UNDP)

The mission of UNDP is to promote sustainable human development and to strengthen international cooperation for sustainable human development. UNDP has a history of promotion of school based health and nutrition approaches. In 1992 it played a leadership role in creating the Partnership for Child Development to undertake operations research into the role of school health and nutrition in child development, and remains a cosponsor.

UNDP is also a cosponsor of the Micronutrient Initiative. UNDP has supported pilot school health and nutrition programmes in Colombia, Ghana, Tanzania, India, Indonesia and Vietnam, and contributed to programmes in some 14 countries. An innovative programme to facilitate the creation of local NGOs in school health and nutrition is being piloted in Africa. UNDP is currently commissioning sector work on development, including an analysis of the role of school-based health and nutrition in child development.

United Nations Population Fund (UNFPA)

UNFPA, along with most of the UN organisations, is increasing the number and scope of health programmes for youth and adolescents. In recognition of the need to strengthen the impetus and direction of actions for adolescent health, WHO, UNFPA and UNICEF jointly convened a Study Group on Programming for Adolescent Health in 1995. This resulted in a number of guidelines for policy direction at the country, regional and global level. Currently, UNFPA support adolescent reproductive health programmes in approximately 100 countries.

These include educational programmes (In-school education programmes can cover population education, family life education, sexuality education, "life-planning" and parent education); information and communication programmes (in-school production of Information, Education and Communication - IEC - materials) and health services programmes. UNFPA also supports HIV/AIDS prevention activities for youth and adolescents in approximately 95 countries within the global strategy of the Joint United Nations Programme on HIV/AIDS (UNAIDS) which became operational in 1996.

The main focus of UNFPA's activities is at the country level where the AIDS prevention activities are integrated into ongoing programmes and projects in reproductive health. Collaboration with NGOs in undertaking HIV/AIDS prevention activities is an integral part of most country programmes. An important objective of many UNFPA programmes is to strengthen the ability of developing countries to carry out the Programme of Action of the International Conference on Population Development (ICPD), agreed by all countries at the conference in 1994.

In Azerbaijan, UNFPA is supporting the Ministry of Education in developing a Family Life Education curriculum in schools (9th, 10th and 11th grades). This addresses issues of STDs, teenage pregnancies and family life/reproduction. In Bhutan, UNFPA supports a programme aimed at increasing accessibility to, and availability of information about, quality reproductive health services, particularly for adolescents.

In China, support for projects that aim to improve access to reproductive health information for adolescents. In Mongolia, support for a Government programme that includes adolescent reproductive health and sexuality education for in-school and out-of-school adolescents.

In Papua New Guinea, UNFPA is providing training to teachers and trainers in incorporating population education into the school curricula. A peer-to-peer counselling centre for adolescent reproductive health has also been established at the University of Papua New Guinea. Women NGOs are also engaged in UNFPA's advocacy activities such as role model visits to schools and reproductive health radio programmes.

In Namibia, UNFPA is supporting the Erongo School Health Initiative, with the local Regional Health Office, WHO and UNICEF. The project aims to improve the knowledge and skills of 90% of learners, by 2005, in prevention of AIDS/HIV/STD/TB, helminth infections and violence. Health education is included in the curriculum and life skills training provided on specific topics such as nutrition, personal hygiene and disease prevention. The programme includes teacher training, provision of school health services, effective monitoring, strengthening of multisectorial involvement and networking in school health programmes. School health services include immunization, screening and referral for sight and hearing problems.

United Nations Programme on HIV/AIDS (UNAIDS)

The United Nations Programme on HIV/AIDS was launched in 1996 and seeks to coordinate global - especially UN - strategy on HIV/AIDS prevention, research and advocacy. Co-sponsors include WHO, UNFPA, UNDP, UNESCO, UNICEF, UNDCP and the World Bank. UNAIDS concentrates on working with all UN Agencies and other partners to comprehensively integrate action on HIV/AIDS. The three areas of focus in UNAIDS activities are:

— *Facilitation of broad action*

— *Advocacy*

— *Identification of best practice in responding to HIV/AIDS*

UNAIDS also acts as an information resource and can provide access to a range of useful materials including; the Best Practice collection, epidemiological information and evaluated materials.

There has been a specific focus on school-based activities, and one of the inter-agency working groups deals only with this topic. The major aim of this group is to promote life skills and Information, Education and Communication about HIV/AIDS programmes through schools.

Although UNAIDS does not have a specific policy towards the school-aged child as such, UNAIDS publishes a range of items that refer to HIV/AIDS prevention for the school-aged child. UNAIDS supports school-based health programmes by facilitating and advocating for action, rather than outright funding. UNAIDS plans and works with UN and other Agencies to advocate for greater attention to HIV prevention. UNAIDS is involved in mobilising partners at the country level, and assisting with technical expertise, as well as developing or attracting the necessary material and human resources to implement programs.

International Atomic Energy Agency (IAEA)

The IAEA has a mandate to enlarge the contribution of atomic energy to health (and peace and prosperity) throughout the world. Specifically, IAEA supports a Human Health Programme, which includes a nutrition and health-related environmental studies sub-programme. Projects supported under this sub-programme include "applied human nutrition assessment and research using nuclear and isotopic techniques" which aims to demonstrate the practical use of nuclear and isotopic techniques as tools for improving nutrition monitoring and for identifying effective food and nutrition strategies in developing countries.

During 1997, the IAEA supported co-ordinated research in 33 developing countries and technical co-operation in 9 countries. Examples of IAEA research programmes include:

— *Peru: Working with the Government on a Model Project which provides food supplements through a daily breakfast to over 500,000 school children over a four year period in six regions of the country. Nuclear techniques are being used to evaluate the programme impact on nutritional status of the school children.*

— *China: Institute of Nutrition and Food Hygiene, Beijing. Project to assess food based intervention of vitamin A status in children (4-6 year olds).*

— *Philippines: Nutrition Centre of the Philippines, Makati City. Project to provide information regarding adequacy of vitamin A measures and efficacy of food-based intervention programs in improving vitamin A status, for children of elementary school age.*

— *Brazil: Ministry of Health, Federal University of Pelotas, University of Sao Paulo. Research project to estimate the effectiveness of the National Programme for Food Assistance of Malnourished Children (milk distribution) on promoting child growth, using isotopic techniques (pre-school children).*

— *Argentina: Ministry of health and CESNI. Research programme to estimate the effectiveness of the Maternal and Child Programme, using isotopic techniques (pre-school and school age children).*

— *Chile: Ministry of Health, INTA, and University of Chile. Research programme to estimate the effectiveness of the National Supplementary Feeding Programme, the National Board of Day Centres, the INTEGRA day-care centres and the School Feeding Programme, using isotopic techniques.*

— *Mexico: Education, Health and Nutrition Program, Mexican Institute of Social Security, and CIAD. Research programme to estimate the effectiveness of the National Nutrition Plan, using isotopic techniques.*

Multilateral Finance Agencies

The World Bank

The World Bank is now giving greater emphasis to

social sector approaches which are child-centred, which target poverty and which are responsive to client country needs. School based health and nutrition programmes contribute to this new approach, and are endorsed in the Health, Nutrition and Population Sector Strategy and are in the current draft of the Education Sector Strategy. Africa Region has a School Health and Nutrition Affinity Group and an articulated strategy.

Latin America and the Caribbean Region also has a strategy paper, and has launched a joint initiative with the Pan American Health Organisation to undertake operations and sector work in the Region. The World Bank is seeking to coordinate information on school health and nutrition approaches through an International School Health Initiative based in the Human Development Network. This seeks to enhance the quality of school health and nutrition programmes by:

- *Providing access to expert advice, particularly in and from client countries.*
- *Providing a clearing house for examples of good practice.*
- *Developing practical toolkits for implementation, based on actual experience.*
- *Making quality information available through the Internet, the World Bank intranet and the World Bank Advisory Services.*
- *Building partnerships with governments and international agencies, institutions and NGOs.*
- *Assisting task teams to prepare school health components for World Bank projects.*

The World Bank has established collaborations in order to promote quality technical input into programme design. The Bank has a formal partnership with PAHO in Latin American Countries (LAC), and is in dialogue with WHO on technical support for Africa. Within the UN system, partnerships are being developed with UNICEF, UNAIDS and WFP, amongst others. Partnerships are also being created with bilaterals.

For example, USAID are co-sponsors of the International School Health Initiative, and DFID, UK, are co-sponsors of sector work on the out of school child. The Bank is also developing partnerships with NGOs, for example Save the Children Federation, USA, and is a co-sponsor of the Partnership for Child Development and the Micronutrient Initiative. The rationale for World Bank interest in school health and nutrition programmes includes the following issues:

— *There are more school-age children, and more in school, than ever before.*

— *School children are neglected by most health systems.*

— *Freedom from disease promotes intellectual as well as physical development.*

— *Healthy children get maximum benefit from their only opportunity for education.*

— *The benefits are greatest for the most disadvantaged - the girl child, the malnourished and the poor.*

— *The combination of an accessible population and an extensive trained workforce of teachers keep financial costs to a minimum.*

— *Builds on the investment in early child development,*

and builds the basics for appropriate social behaviour in adolescence.

Experiences of good practice suggest that, in terms of World Bank Human Development strategy, school-based health and nutrition programmes should be simple and locally relevant, and should not overload already overstretched teachers or the curriculum. The following items might usefully contribute to such programmes:

— *Life Skills Training and IEC - as part of a strategy to promote healthy lifestyles, and avoid violence, substance abuse, HIV/AIDS and teenage pregnancy.*

— *Health Services - as part of the Primary Health Care system, and providing screening for sight and hearing, simple health interventions (deworming, first aid) and referral.*

— *School Snacks - which are fortified with micronutrients and provided early in the school day.*

— *Exemplary School Environment - which supports health education messages about hygiene and sanitation.*

— *Equitable School Health Policies - that ensure the rights of school children.*

— *Strategies Beyond the School - that use the school as a community centre to provide services to out of school children.*

A Knowledge Management Site has been established on the intranet to assist World Bank task teams to prepare school health and nutrition components for client governments. As part of the International School Health Initiative this site is being transferred to the external internet, where it will be supported by a mail list for exchange of information amongst co-sponsors and subscribers. The activities described above are intended to build and promote partnerships with technical agencies and to ensure the quality of technical advice to client governments. Bank operations in school health and nutrition involve the inclusion of this component within government projects or sector-wide approaches supported by Bank credit.

Inter-American Development Bank (IADB)

The Inter-American Development Bank, the oldest and largest regional multilateral development institution, was established in 1959 to help accelerate economic and social development in Latin America and the Caribbean. The Bank's operations cover the entire spectrum of economic and social development, including public health and education.

Current lending priorities include the areas of poverty reduction, social equity, modernisation and integration. IADB has an established record in supporting school-based health and nutrition projects. In El Salvador the "Basic Education Modernisation" project aims to promote greater equity, quality and efficiency in the provision of education services. The components include activities to develop a school health and nutrition programme targeted to the El Salvador's poorest 135 municipalities. The total resources allocated are US $1.5 million. Other donors to this project include the World Bank.

In Mexico, the "Integrated Compensatory Education Programme" has a number of aims which include increasing access to education among poor children, providing child-rearing education to illiterate/ uneducated parents, literacy training for adults and education in remote areas without schools. Specifically, parents are trained to recognise the imperative of good nutrition in fostering healthy growth and development. They are also taught how to improve nutrition and developmental activities.

In Jamaica, the "Primary Education Improvement Programme II" supports research into the link between cognition and nutrition to enable the Ministry of Education to plan the timing and distribution of its nutri-bun programme.

Asian Development Bank (ADB)

The ADB emphasises its strategic objective of promoting human development by expanding investments in the critical sectors of education, health and nutrition, water supply and sanitation. School health programmes supported by the ADB include:

— *Nepal:* *Assistance to Primary School Feeding, in collaboration with WHO and bilateral donors. The project aims to enhance learning capacity by alleviating short-term hunger and to reduce the prevalence and intensity of intestinal parasites by deworming.*

— *Kyrgyz Republic:* *Community-Based Early Childhood Development. This projects includes a package of nutrition interventions such as community -and- school level growth monitoring and food supplementation interventions to address micronutrient and protein/energy deficiencies.*

— *Pakistan: Primary School Quality Improvement. This project includes the provision of free textbooks, incentives to keep girls in school and special courses in nutrition and life skills. It also provides interventions to upgrade shelterless schools (schools without roof or wall).*

Bilateral Organisations

Canadian International Development Agency (CIDA)

CIDA is a lead donor in the area of nutrition programming. Since 1992, CIDA has contributed over $87 million to nutrition projects of which $78 million have been focused on micronutrients. An additional $120 million has been contributed to integrated projects which combine nutrition with health, basic education and income generation activities. CIDA is a founding member of the Micronutrient Initiative (MI) which has a grant of approximately $53 million and is supported by IDRC, UNDP, UNICEF, USAID and the World Bank.

Although CIDA's budget is not exclusively channelled through the school system, examples of CIDA programmes that affect the school-aged child include:

— *Funding to WFP for school feeding/health programmes and through the Women's Health Facility.*

— *The MI South Asia Programme which aims to eliminate iodine and vitamin A deficiency and reduce iron deficiency in women in Bangladesh, India, Nepal and Pakistan by the year 2000.*

— *The Ecuador Iodine Deficiency Disorder (IDD) Programme which has implemented a school-based IDD monitoring system where school children bring samples of salt to school to test for iodine in class using low-cost rapid tests.*

— *A School Feeding Programme in Haiti implemented by a French-Canadian NGO costing $1.6 million which started in 1998.*

CIDA recognises the link between girls' education wider health issues, and that discrimination against the education of girls is an important area to address in many countries. "Women's education, especially the number of years of schooling, is closely related to reduction of child mortality and morbidity , improvement of family health and nutrition, and decline in population growth."

CIDA (with UNICEF) supports a programme for the advancement of girls' education in Zambia, providing equipment, services, advisors and trainees. The aim is to increase capacity at all levels and to improve rates of enrolment, retention, completion and achievement of primary school girls.

In Egypt CIDA, with UNICEF, supports the development of management and technical capacity for sustaining a community-based, girl-friendly education model. CIDA also supports the Egyptian Government's program for opening 3000 new one room schools. CIDA's support for programmes that increase access to education also includes Non Formal Primary Education in Bangladesh, aimed at providing cost effective primary education for children, particularly girls, who are outside the formal education system.

This programme is co-funded by the Aga Khan Foundation Canada. CIDA also supports the Adolescent Development Program in Bangladesh, that aims to improve the future economic and social status of adolescent girls by providing them with literacy, numeracy, health education and income earning skills. CIDA are also involved in support of basic primary health care in many countries, Roll Back Malaria campaigns, STOP TB initiative and HIV/AIDS programming in many regions of the world.

Danish International Development Assistance (DANIDA)

DANIDA do not have a defined strategy for support towards school based health programmes although they are supporting other agencies through their bilateral programme. For example funding to UNICEF in Uganda for school based health education activities. Members of the education and health sector in DANIDA have discussed the need for school-based health and nutrition programming on a number of occasions but constraints on time and finances have prevented them from taking this further.

Although DANIDA's water and sanitation strategy, "Water, Sanitation and Hygiene (WASH)" does not refer to schoolchildren directly, DANIDA supports the provision of water supplies to primary schools within their rural water supplies programmes in developing countries. The health education component of their water strategy, which incorporates messages about hygiene behaviour and water-related diseases also, targets primary schools.

Department for International Development of U.K. (DFID)

DFID do not have a current policy which refers specifically to the school aged child although they have supported a range of projects and programmes which directly benefit this group. In Bolivia, a reproductive health project for adolescents which includes curriculum development, development of teacher training materials and teacher training systems targeted at 13 year olds. Also in Bolivia, DFID support a project that aims to improve the living conditions of school children through health education as an integral part of the school curriculum. An example of this is a project to increase awareness about Chagas disease using health education in schools as well as radio broadcasts.

In India, DFID have supported a large programme in Andhra Pradesh aimed at improving the health of school children by reorganising and strengthening existing school health services. The programme, costing more than UKPDS 4 million over a five-year period has recently been terminated for diverse reasons.

Also in India DFID provides funding for the School Health Action and training Programme (SeHAT) Programme and its expansion into Delhi centre (see Child to Child and AHRTAG). In Iraq, the rehabilitation of school facilities, water and sanitation systems and the procurement and distribution of educational materials in order to prevent the spread of communicable diseases in the schools.

In Kenya, HIV/AIDS prevention for the 7 - 14 year age group and a project that supports low-cost rainwater catchment tanks for 800 schools in 8 districts with an estimated coverage of 300,000 children. In Mozambique, DFID supports SCF to promote the integration of disabled school children into mainstream school.

In Peru, support is given to the work of the United Nations Drug Control Programme (UNCDP) on drug abuse prevention through primary education curriculum development and teacher training. DFID also support many countries HIV/AIDS Control Programmes that target school-aged children.

Norwegian Agency for Development Co-operation (NORAD)

NORAD does not have a particular policy focus for school-aged children but does support the education sectors in many developing countries in basic education programmes, including teacher training (e.g. Eritrea, Tanzania, Nepal) greater access to education for girls (e.g. Ethiopia, Uganda, Zambia, Mali, Bangladesh) and construction of schools (e.g. Palestine). In Malawi NORAD provides assistance through the reform programme "Keeping Kids in School", which is coordinated by UNICEF.

Under this programme, which targets children from first to fourth grade in primary school, 18 new schools were built and 76 teachers trained in 1998. The programme also includes providing water supplies and digging hygienic latrines on school sites, with associated education in hygiene and simple health precautions.

NORAD are currently supporting a School Nutrition Programme (SNP) in Sindh, Pakistan which is implemented with co-operation from the Government of Sindh and Aga Khan University along with NGOs.

The SNP is a pilot programme that supports school feeding in schools in four rural districts. Initiated in 1994 the programme reaches around 12,000 beneficiaries and supports the following objectives:

- *Increase enrolment, retention and regular attendance of children, especially girls, in school*
- *Improve the nutritional status of primary school children and their siblings*
- *Improve student achievement*
- *Increase parental and community awareness of the importance of child nutrition and education*
- *Explore possibilities for community involvement at the school level in improving education and nutrition*
- *Explore the possibilities for implementing SNP through NGOs.*

The SNP supports participatory training for PTAs and NGOs to enable them to take increasing responsibility for the programme and thus ensure its long-term sustainability. PTAs are responsible for dealing with the funds, food purchasing and in some areas, food preparation. The formation and commitment of the PTAs is viewed as a particular strength of the programme.

The SNP is being expanded into additional districts and is being considered as an approach for replication in Nepal. The impact of the SNP has recently been evaluated which suggests that whilst the nutritional status of children has improved along with the school enrolment and retention rates, there has also been a decline in educational achievement.

The latter may be due to the programme demands on parents and children time. NORAD works closely with relevant UN agencies (such as UNICEF) and with NGOs, including both national organisations in the country where specific programmes are in operation and with international NGOs where appropriate.

Swedish International Development Agency (SIDA)

SIDA has no special policy with respect to the health and nutrition of the school aged child but supports basic education and education reform. Within their education reform programme, SIDA supports, and intend to increase their support for, curriculum development work relating to HIV/AIDS education such as the production of materials, teacher training and the use of popular theatre media etc to reduce risk behaviour.

They consider school-based programmes to be most effective if integrated with other curriculum content i.e. health education, social science and biology. They are working closely with governments as well as international organisations (UNAIDS and UNICEF) and NGOs. They also support UNESCO's resource centre for HIV/AIDS education and UNESCO's regional training programme for HIV/AIDS education.

The importance of sexual and reproductive health is acknowledged by SIDA in its "Strategy for Promotion of Sexual and Reproductive Health and Rights in Development Cooperation". This strategy addresses key issues such as abortion, fertility regulation, prevention and control of STDs, including HIV. Specific emphasis is placed on adolescents' sexual and reproductive health.

SIDA sees peer education programmes as particularly important in this area. An emphasis on gender equality is also seen as important. SIDA and NORAD are co-funding an African Medical Research Foundation (AMREF) project "Regional Adolescent Sexual and Reproductive Health (ASHR) Project" with components in Kenya, Tanzania, Uganda and Ethiopia.

The project aims to "achieve an improved and maintained health status of adolescents in the region through healthy sexual relations and behaviour, reduced exposure to STD/HIV, unwanted pregnancy and increased access to effective services". Youth both in and out of school are targeted as well as service providers, teachers, parents and community elders. In the broader area of child health in general, SIDA places emphasis on preventive measures (e.g. immunisation) and on the integrated management of childhood illness.

United States Agency for International Development (USAID)

USAID is the United States federal government agency that implements America's foreign economic and humanitarian assistance programs. USAID's Africa Bureau (Office of Sustainable Development/Education) has formulated a school health position paper that emphasises the same program elements and rationale as that of the World Bank.

USAID's position paper particularly emphasises

that school health activities should support education systems reform, and it emphasises community mobilisation for support of pupil nutrition and community cost-sharing for school-based health interventions. These emphases aim to maximise community impact of health interventions and education, and program sustainability. USAID's Africa Bureau is also a co-sponsor of the International School Health Initiative based at the World Bank.

USAID support large school-based health programs that deliver health interventions such as deworming and micronutrient supplementation across Africa. Many of these programs are in various stages of evaluation. USAID also support smaller school health activities such as latrine construction, community based nutrition grants, school gardens and borehole drilling within USAID and UNICEF sponsored programmes in Africa.

Civil Society; Non-Governmental Organisations (NGOs)

ActionAid

ActionAid works in countries in Africa and Asia and Latin America. 60% of their income is provided by child sponsors who regularly contribute to projects. Other sources of income include appeals, grants from the UK National Lottery Charity Board and Comic Relief. Support is given in a number of areas such as: emergency relief projects; health - particularly maternal and child; education - including adult literacy, increasing access to education, renovating and building schools; water and sanitation; HIV/AIDS prevention.

The Aga Khan Foundation (AKF)

Over the last fifteen years, the Aga Khan Foundation has supported various programmes in the area of health education, particularly in six countries: India, Tanzania (Zanzibar), Pakistan, Uganda, Kenya and, most recently, Tajikistan. AKF also supported the Child-to-Child Trust in the United Kingdom during its early years. The AKF-funded health education projects have usually followed the Child-to-Child approach, aiming to increase the knowledge and practices of good health promoting behaviours in school-aged children: i.e., Informed children pass on key health messages and practices to their peers and younger children and also share the information with their families and the wider community.

When AKF developed its Education Programme, it included attention to the importance of early childhood development and school improvement at primary and secondary levels. AKF supports programmes which recognize that children are part of a family and wider community which influence, and are influenced by, them (the children). The average duration of AKF funding for education projects is six years.

This has generally been enough time to experiment with a curriculum model and make changes, develop training and support materials, begin to disseminate the results, and assist the project in becoming self-sufficient. For example, one of the first Child-to-Child projects in Delhi, India become the basis for a national health education programme sponsored by the government.

Americna Jewish World Service (AJWS)

Founded in 1985, AJWS provides non-sectarian humanitarian assistance to disadvantaged people in Africa, Asia, Latin America, the Middle East, Russia and Ukraine. Working in partnership with local grassroots NGOs, AJWS supports and implements small-scale international development projects.

Healthlink Worldwide

Although Healthlink Worldwide has no formal policy or guidelines on school health, they support school-based health programmes through both programming and funding. The main focus of Healthlink Worldwide's support for school age children is in the area of health education, producing educational materials for use by school children, and using innovative approaches for training teachers in the use of these materials. The emphasis is on general health and nutrition, although this may include educational and promotional work in areas such as HIV/AIDS, water and sanitation.

Healthlink Worldwide is supporting the Municipal Corporation of Delhi and Bombay Municipal Corporation, through an NGO called SEARCH New Delhi (Society for Education Action and Research in Community Health) to implement one large programme in India that focuses on primary schools in Delhi and Bombay called the School Health Action and Training Project (SeHAT). SeHAT received funding from, DFID, European Union, UK National Lottery Charity Fund, Stanley Thomas Johnson Foundation and the Aga Khan Foundation.

Initially Healthlink Worldwide and the School

Health Services in Delhi ran a pilot programme in selected low-income schools for four years, developing methods and materials for incorporating health topics into the curriculum. These include communicable diseases, sanitation, nutrition and personal cleanliness as well as other health-related behaviour including tobacco, safety and pollution.

Government policy informs the programme approach: a re-orientation of teaching methodology away from traditional didactic techniques and towards child-centred, activity based teaching that fosters informed choice and a teacher-led, curriculum oriented approach to health education in schools.

Healthlink Worldwide is currently exploring ways of incorporating malaria education and control into health promoting schools in Sub Saharan Africa, in collaboration with the Malaria Consortium, the London School of Tropical Medicine and the Liverpool School of Tropical Medicine. Other plans include collaboration with the Child to Child Trust in a project working with families affected by HIV/AIDS in Kenya and Uganda, involving both school age children and development of children under five.

Care

Care has a number of program areas that affect school-aged children, these include:

— *Education - promoting literacy, numeracy, and school attendance, especially among girls.*

— *Food Security - including school feeding.*

— *Health and Population - encompassing promotion of*

> *AIDS awareness and prevention, children's health, water and sanitation. CARE integrates reproductive health efforts with other programmes, including girls' education, water and sanitation, microenterprise and children's health.*

Care supports a range of school health and nutrition projects through its education and health programmes.

In Thailand, the Children's Health and Environment magazine Project produces and distributes a cartoon-format children's magazine that teaches primary school children about health and environmental issues. Each edition is distributed to 31,000 schools countrywide and is read by over 1 million students. The project also provides a teacher's guide and seeks to inform and motivate students so that they can positively influence environmental practices and community health.

In Kenya, CARE supports health education in schools using Child to Child approaches and school based water and sanitation clubs.

In Laos, CARE supports a school nutrition project which involves community based activities for all the primary schools in 22 villages (planting fruit trees and establishing vegetable gardens, fisheries and poultry farming).

In Zambia, they support peri-urban schools for children who are HIV/AIDS orphans.

Catholic Fund for Overseas Development (CAFOD)

CAFOD's current guidelines are not to support formal education. Recently, however, they are reconsidering their policy on this as Asian and African governments are increasingly requesting assistance in the education sector (including health and nutrition). This has prompted an analysis of the issues in CAFOD who have been developing a database of existing education-based programmes, which is now nearing completion.

CAFOD support a range of small programmes in Africa and Asia (usually through partners) that affect the school age child but are not school-based. Examples include support for orphans of AIDS victims through the provision of school fees and education materials; youth programmes which include health components, for example HIV/AIDS education and life skills training.

Caribbean Food and Nutrition Institute (CFNI)

CFNI have supported two studies relating to school aged children: Nutrition Education and the Consumption of Fruits and Vegetables in School Children and After School Physical Activity Programme and Academic Performance and Fitness Levels of Jamaican Adolescents.

Catholic Relief Services (CRS)

CRS is currently implementing/supporting education programming in approximately 25 countries in Africa, Asia, Europe/Balkans, Latin America, and the Caribbean. Of these, approximately 15 country programs are implementing health/hygiene/nutrition (HHN) programming within schools or nonformal education settings. Twelve of these 15 are carrying out school feeding programs. Of the school feeding programs, most (Burkina Faso, Ghana, Liberia, Sierra Leone, Benin, Sudan, Haiti, India) are being funded primarily by USAID's Food for Peace office. Another three are funded by the European Community (Pakistan, Egypt, Armenia), and one (Mali) is funded by World Food Programme.

In addition, Egypt is implementing a nonformal education program for adolescent girls which has a large health education component, funded by CEDPA (Centre for Education, Development, & Population Activities). Most of the CRS-supported school health activities are not stand-alone projects but rather are integrated with other project activities which focus on improving education access, quality, and achievement.

Child to Child Trust (CTC)

CtC support child centred approaches to health education through:

— *Design and distribution of health education materials which are used by children, teachers and health workers.*

– *Advice and assistance to health education workers in planning, implementing and evaluating projects using the Child-to Child approach.*

— *Coordinating a Worldwide information network for people and projects around the world who use the Child-to-Child approach.*

The school based approach is undertaken in-line with the WHO Global Initiative and emphasises what poorer schools can realistically do to improve the health of school children within the framework of existing resources and without the exploitation of children or the over-burdening of the teachers.

Priority areas for the Child-to-Child Trust are:

— Helping children who live in difficult circumstances, for example those who live in refugee camps, children affected by war, and children with disabilities.

— Improving health promotion in schools, involving children in spreading good health ideas and practices to families, out-of-school children and the wider community.

— Supporting the development of local Child-to-Child resource units and networks.

In Pakistan, a five year pilot project entitled Health Action Schools Pilot Project has been initiated to develop prototypes for 'Health Action' schools and is funded by the Aga Khan Foundation and SCF UK. The project, which is located in contrasting socio-economic areas (urban, rural and mixed urban/rural) supports the development of training and support networks for schools endeavouring to become 'Health Action' schools and has an operational research component to identify changes in health awareness, health behaviour and education performance among the school children.

In Kenya, a CtC project has been implemented through which it is hoped that major policy changes will occur, especially the inclusion of health education as a separate curriculum subject in primary education. The programme, based on a three-year plan supports the dissemination of CtC; training for those working for

'Health Action' schools, production of materials, and teacher training in CtC. Funding is provided by DANIDA.

CtC resource units and networks have been developed to promote and encourage Child-to-Child activities in the Arab world, Central and South America, East and West Africa and India.

Christian Aid (CA)

Christian Aid works in over 60 countries throughout the world. It runs emergency appeals for areas in crisis. It campaigns for fair trade and an end to Third World Debt and has highlighted issues such as the child sex industry in southeast Asia and child labour in Pakistan.

Educating children on health issues through the existing school system. An example of this support is the 'Molo Songololo' project in South Africa which works with school-age children on children's rights and the promotion of equity among all races to promote a more equal society. Molo publish a magazine that is read by more than 50,000 children and teachers.

Also in South Africa, CA supports the African and Educational Puppetry Production (AREPP) which focuses on HIV/AIDS awareness, children's empowerment which tackles issues around child abuse. These productions are performed throughout SA in urban and rural schools.

Helen Keller International (HKI)

From 1982 to the present, a significant increase in

USAID and private funding has allowed HKI to accelerate its program development and expand in to new countries in Africa and South America. Staff have increased to include specialists in several areas: paediatrics, optometry, ophthalmology, research, evaluation, trachoma, cataract surgery, public health and service delivery, epidemiology, training and health education, operations research, microcredit, water and sanitation, surveillance, operations research, nutrition, and onchocerciasis.

Technical assistance is provided through a partnership role with governments and local organisations. All partnerships are developed with the expectation of eventual HKI withdrawal based on a turnover of responsibility within a given period. The primary goal of HKI programs has become upgrading local and indigenous skills in areas of service delivery, program design and implementation, evaluation, and operations research.

HKI does not have policy towards school-age children as such, but is developing programs for this age group. Support for programmes that are school based is generally in the form of pilot projects, but may include operations research (e.g. a project in Indonesia).

HKI also supports programmes that include health education about use of latrines, face washing (for trachoma prevention) and use of clean water. Trachoma initiatives, aimed at children from 5 - 11 years, are planned for Mali, Niger, Tanzania, Morocco, Burkina Faso, Mozambique and Nepal.

Oxfam

Oxfam is currently running a campaign in education. The campaign on education is aimed at achieving national and international policy changes to contribute to the goal of universal primary education by 2015. Oxfam has education programmes in several countries in Africa, South Asia and Latin America.

The aim is to scale up these programmes as part of Oxfam contribution to the education for all objective. Although there is no specific health aspect at present, these programmes are building a framework where health education could be introduced in the future. Oxfam are also interested in collaborating with other organisations in the delivery of school health interventions.

Partnership for Child Development (PCD)

The Partnership for Child Development was set up in 1992 to undertake operations research on school health programmes. The Partnership is involved in research, technical advice and support in some 50 countries throughout the world. The Partnership tests and evaluates simple, low cost school health programmes in several countries at an operationally realistic scale, involving between 50,000 and 3 million children in widely scattered sites throughout the world.

Peace Corps

The Peace Corps was established in the USA in 1961. It is a voluntary organisation with approximately 155,00 volunteers working on development projects in 134 countries around the world. 40% of volunteers work in education and 18% in health. Both these fields include projects with school health components.

Peace Corps education projects often seek to improve education for women and girls. They include primary education projects with a particular focus on health education and awareness. Health Extension volunteers aim to raise consciousness in communities about the need for health education. They may also assist in the training of trainers for peer education about STDs/AIDS. An example of a Peace Corps program in the area of AIDS prevention is the 'Teach English Prevent AIDS' program in Cameroon, which involves the teaching of English in Francophone schools, using health education about HIV/AIDS prevention.

Water and Sanitation Extension Volunteers serve in a broad range of water/sanitation projects and hygiene education activities. This includes constructing wells, tapping springs and building latrines; improving facilities for storing potable water and doing community outreach to heighten awareness of water, sanitation and health issues.

Plan International (PLAN)

PLAN is one of the world's largest child-focused development organisations. PLAN has five main inter-related "Domain and Programme Principles";

— *Growing up Healthy*

— *Learning*

— *Habitat*

— *Livelihood*

— *Building Relations.*

PLAN's Growing up Healthy Domain is concerned with the physical and mental health of children, that of

2

Health and Nutrition of School-age Child

Children of school age face health and nutrition problems that may affect their individual physical development, their capacity to attend school and their ability to learn. The aetiology of impaired cognitive development is now a central area for concern while improvements in cognitive performance produce opportunities for evaluating the impact of school health and nutrition programmes.

The situation of school-age children who do not attend school is reviewed separately. There is growing concern that non-school attenders may suffer disproportionately from ill health and malnutrition and that these insults may continue through their primary school years. In other words, non-attendance at school is both a symptom and a cause of multiple deprivation. The main nutritional problems facing the school-age child include stunting, underweight, anaemia and iodine deficiency and, on the basis of information from recent surveys, vitamin A deficiency may also be an important problem in this age group.

In countries experiencing the 'nutrition transition', overweight and obesity are growing problems in the school-age child. The main health problems facing school-age children are helminth infections, malaria, diarrhoeal diseases, respiratory infections and tuberculosis. Much of the disease burden derives from the poor environmental conditions in which they live including exposure to biological, chemical and physical hazards in the environment and a lack of resources essential for human health.

Malnutrition

Stunting (low height-for-age) and underweight (low weight-for-age) are widespread problems in developing countries and can reflect a broad range of insults such as prenatal undernutrition, deficiencies of macronutrients and micronutrients, infection and, possibly, inadequate attention by caregivers. The cause of stunting is widely believed to occur mainly in early childhood through a cumulative process. Stunting is known to be important in young children because it can have long-term consequences for entry into school, learning, educational performance and productivity.

It is also associated in females with negative outcomes for future pregnancies. In spite of this, there has been relatively little information gathered on the nutritional status of the school-age child and this is reflected in the lack of clear guidelines for assessing their growth and the functional significance of various threshold points for assessing their nutritional status.

Variation in the rate of maturation and growth make the interpretation of adolescent growth patterns particularly difficult.

The WHO Expert Committee on Anthropometry recommends that physical measurement of adolescents should be accompanied by puberty status assessment to properly interpret growth in this age group. Identifying the timing of puberty in different populations, however, is often difficult. Overall, boys tend to experience the adolescent growth spurt later than girls and are likely to have a greater growth potential than girls.

New information that is emerging from the most recent studies into the nutritional status of school-age children strongly suggest that school-age children suffer from higher levels of undernutrition than have been previously acknowledged. This is particularly true in the case of stunting which is increasingly being used as an indicator of population well being and an indicator for poverty. The degree and prevalence of stunting and underweight have been found to increase with age with older children diverging further from the reference medians for height.

The increased degree and prevalence of stunting with age could be explained by the delayed onset of puberty in both boys and girls. It also appears, however, that although children show evidence of growth into late adolescence, that full 'catch-up' growth is not occurring but that linear growth retardation persists throughout the primary school years. These findings are contrary to the formerly widely held view that stunting is a process that usually happens in early childhood. Boys are more likely to be stunted and underweight than girls.

In some countries, boys were also significantly more likely to be wasted or thin than girls. The reason for the apparent higher levels of stunting in boys is unclear and may be influenced by a bias in the school population. It is also suggested that it could reflect delayed onset of puberty, itself caused by undernutrition and the failure to reach their growth potential through slow compensatory linear growth.

One of the largest and most recent studies into the anthropometric status of rural schoolchildren in developing countries has been carried out in West and East Africa, in South and North Asia and the Indian subcontinent. Three important findings were generated from this work. First, the overall prevalence of stunting and underweight was found to be high in all five countries, ranging from 48-56% for stunting and from 34 and 62% for underweight. The prevalence of wasting was found to be particularly high in Vietnam and India affecting 21 and 31% of children respectively but was much less common than stunting or underweight in the other three countries. Children in Vietnam and India also showed higher levels of underweight and stunting than children in the other three countries.

Second, in all countries there was a trend for z-scores of height-for-age and weight-for-age to decrease with age, thus as children got older they became shorter than the reference population. This suggests that either younger children are better nourished than the older children are and therefore that nutrition is improving in all five countries or, that linear growth deficits are persisting throughout the school-age years.

Third, boys in most countries tended to be significantly more stunted than girls and in all countries boys were more underweight than girls. A higher drop out rate of girls than boys may explain this although in two of the countries, the sex ratios in classes were equal. An alternative explanation is that the adolescent growth spurt is either delayed in boys or is not occurring at all. A distinct growth-spurt was not identified in either girls or boys although linear growth did persist into the late teens, beyond the years usually associated with growth in puberty.

One of the few longitudinal studies of changes in height and weight of school-age children has been conducted on Pemba Island, Zanzibar over a period of one year. The findings are remarkably similar to those found in the study described above with growth in height continuing to diverge from the reference values as age increases.

In Chile, a country undergoing the nutrition transition, height deficits have been compared among children entering first grade in 1987, 1990, 1993 and 1996. Overall, height deficits have declined in both boys and girls although the overall height deficit in boys was found to be greater in each period studied. A recent cross-sectional survey of the nutritional status of adolescent boys and girls in Bangladesh found that 67% of adolescents were thin and 48% were stunted. Whereas thinness was found to decline in prevalence with age from 95% at age 10 years to 12% at age 17years, the prevalence of stunting increased.

Overall the prevalence of stunting was 48% and this rose from 34% at age ten years to 65% at age 17 years. 77% of boys were found to be stunted by the age of 17 years compared to 34% of girls at the same age. Boys were also more likely to be thin than girls. A study into the gender differences in growth of school-age children with helminth infections in Brazil found that 21% of school-age children were stunted and 13% were underweight.

Studies in Latin America and the Caribbean have found that the prevalence of stunting among first grade school children, is higher in rural than in urban communities. This probably reflects the differential access to livelihoods and services in the two areas. Deficiencies of iron, iodine and vitamin A are a major problem in developing countries. Micronutrient deficiencies can negatively effect the mental development and learning ability of schoolchildren and increase their susceptibility to infection.

Iron deficiency and anaemia

Iron deficiency (ID) is the most common nutritional disorder in the world and is estimated to affect more than 2 billion people of whom 1.2 billion suffer from iron deficiency anaemia (IDA) It is estimated that 210 million school-age children suffer from IDA. The main focus of IDA reduction programmes has been on young children and women of reproductive age because of the increased risk of postpartum and perinatal mortality, intrauterine growth retardation and low birth-weight. Insufficient intake of iron rich foods is the major cause of ID. It can also be caused by parasitic infections and deficiencies of other nutrients.

There is substantial evidence that IDA in children is associated with decreased physical and mental development and impaired immune function. Iodine deficiency affects an estimated 1.6 billion people worldwide and an estimated 60 million school-age children. The consequences of iodine deficiency, collectively referred to as iodine deficiency disorders (IDD), include severe mental retardation, goitre, abortion, stillbirths and low birth weight and mild forms of motor and cognitive deficits. Adolescent girls are an important target group for IDD control because of the adverse consequences on foetal development of iodine deficiency during pregnancy and because they generally have a higher prevalence of goitre than boys.

Vitamin A deficiency is widely recognised as an important cause of blindness in children. Mild or sub-clinical vitamin A deficiency causes impaired immune function and, an increased risk of mortality from infectious diseases that can have an effect on school attendance and consequently academic performance. It is estimated that 85 million school-age children are at increased risk of acute respiratory and other infections because they are deficient in vitamin A.

Vitamin A deficiency also affects iron metabolism so that with any iron supplements taken, subsequent improvement in iron status may be limited when vitamin A status is low. This is being increasingly recognised as a potential constraint when considering the impact of school-based iron supplementation.

There are a number of new studies that emphasise the high prevalence of iron deficiency and anaemia in school-age children. These provide further justification for the current focus on providing iron supplements to schoolchildren in areas of high prevalence. Younger children appear to have lower haemoglobin concentrations than older children while older children have a higher prevalence of anaemia. Differences between the sexes do not appear to be significant.

In a survey of nearly 13,000 rural schoolchildren in Africa and Asia, the prevalence of IDA was more than 40% in 6 African countries among children aged 7-11 years and in 4 African countries among children aged 12-14 years. In the 2 Asian countries studied, the overall prevalence of IDA was found to be considerably lower than in Africa. Children aged 7-11 years were found to have lower mean haemoglobin concentrations, while IDA was found to be more common in the older age group.

Girls were also found to have lower haemoglobin concentrations than boys, although the overall prevalence of IDA was higher in boys, particularly in the 12-13 year age group. An in-depth survey of 2,998 children aged 8-9 and 12-13 years in Ghana and Tanzania revealed that 77% of children in Tanzania and 41% of children in Ghana were suffering from IDA. Overall, the mean haemoglobin concentration was lower in the 8-9 year olds and in Ghana, IDA was also more common in the younger age group.

In a study of adolescent males and females in Bangladesh, extremely high levels of anaemia were identified in both females and males. More males were found to be suffering from IDA at a younger age than females whereas females remained very anaemic throughout their adolescence.

School-age children are often used to assess IDD because of their physiological vulnerability and their accessibility through schools. The measurement of goitre in school-age children is important because it can be used to reflect the current status of IDD in the general population. In a recent study of school-age children suffering from mild and moderate iodine deficiency in

Bangladesh, it was found that hypothyroid children performed worse than euthyroid children for reading and spelling

A recent study of school children in Egypt found an overall prevalence rate of goitre of 34.6% indicating a severe public health problem. In Swaziland, nearly half of the schoolchildren surveyed were found to be iodine deficient and 13% were at risk from severe IDD. In South Africa, prior to universal salt iodization, a total goitre prevalence rate of over 70% was found in primary school children from one district confirming severe iodine deficiency.

Short-term hunger

In addition to the problems associated with malnutrition in school-age children, there is also evidence of negative consequences for children suffering from short-term hunger, common in children who are not fed before going to school. Children who are hungry are more likely to have difficulty concentrating and performing complex tasks, even if otherwise well nourished.

Overweight and Obesity

Overweight and obesity is becoming increasingly prevalent in developing countries where improvements in socio-economic conditions and rapid urbanisation are causing a 'nutrition transition'. This is characterised by a rapid shift in the composition of diet (higher fat and lower carbohydrate), (reduced) activity patterns and a subsequent shift in body composition. In emerging economies, levels of childhood overweight and obesity are reported to be rising to levels reported in the United

States.

Stunting is also believed to be a risk factor for obesity and it is suggested that this relationship may lead to considerable problems with obesity in children in developing countries over the coming decades. Chile, which has undergone a major epidemiological and nutrition transition over the past few decades, has a growing problem of overweight and obesity, in adults and in children. A study of school-age children in four countries undergoing the nutrition transition found that the prevalence of child overweight ranged from 10.5% to 25.6%.

Health status is now accepted as a proxy indicator for poverty. The poor, particularly children in developing countries, carry the greatest burden of morbidity and mortality. Much of this burden results from hazards within their homes or their immediate environment. High levels of malnutrition, and its known synergistic relationship exacerbate their vulnerability to disease particularly diarrhoeal disease, ARIs and malaria.

For the urban poor in developing countries, there is a double jeopardy as they find themselves exposed to both "traditional" diseases of poor sanitation and overcrowding and the "modern" diseases of chronic heart and lung disease. School-age children living in poor urban areas are also at a high risk of injury from road traffic accidents.

Intestinal parasitic helminth infections are a major public health problem throughout the world. Prevalence is estimated at 1 billion for ascariasis, 900 million for trichuriasis, 500 million for hookworm and 200 million for schistosomiasis. School-age children are the most heavily infected group both in terms of prevalence and intensity of infection. Helminth infections are estimated to account for over 12% of the total disease burden in girls aged 5 to 14 years and over 11% of the burden in boys making this the single largest contributor to the disease burden of this group.

Obesity is defined as an excessive accumulation of body fat. How much fat is "excessive" depends on the height and weight of the child. Between 5%-25% of children and teenagers in the United States are obese. The prevalence of obesity in the young varies by ethnic group. It is esti-mated that 5%-7% of Caucasian and African-American children are obese while 12% of Hispanic boys and 19% of Hispanic girls are obese. Studies show an alarming rise in obesity among children in the United States during the past twenty years.

Not all obese infants become obese children, and not all obese children become obese adults. However, the prevalence of obesity increases with age among both males and females and it is more likely that obese adolescents will be become obese adults. Obesity presents numerous problems for the child. It takes a toll both in physical health and psycho-social adjustment.

Childhood obesity is the leading cause of pediatric hypertension, is associated with Type II diabetes mellitus, increases the risk of coronary heart disease and increases stress on the weight-bearing joints. Studies have shown that obese children receive less acceptance from their peers and more discrimination from significant adults in their lives, exhibit a greater sense of rejection and failure, have poorer interpersonal relationships, and have limited group and social interests.

Childhood obesity most likely results from an interaction of nutritional, psychological, familial and physiological factors. The risk of becoming obese is greatest among children who have two obese parents. Although there is controversy around how much genetic factors play into obesity, parental modeling of both eating and exercise behaviors affects the children.

In children, underactivity is a significant source of obesity, and as they grow older their activity levels decrease further. In general, weight loss diets are not recommended for most children. Not only is this approach psychologically stressful, but it may adversely affect growth and the child's perception of normal eating.

A child's well-being and adopting a healthy eating and exercise style are more important than pounds lost. Successful behavioral strategies show considerable success in effect-ing long-term weight loss in both handicapped and nonhanicapped children. The best programs incorporate an exercise component and nutritional training, including slowing the rate of eating, limiting the time and place of eating, and problem solving exercises. Particularly effective are behav-iorally based treatments that involve parents.

Obesity is easier to prevent than to treat. Starting in early childhood, teach children proper nutrition, selection of low-fat snacks, good exercise/activity habits and monitor their television viewing. Make good nutrition and exercise a family affair by planning lower fat meals, nutritious snacks and family activities.

This makes the child feel included in a total family effort focused and health and not the isolated one with the problem. Do not use food as a reward for an accomplishment, a substitute for love or compensation for a disappointment.

Teach children to recognize how their body tells them that they are hungry or full. Encourage children to eat a wide variety of foods in moderation. Do not encourage continued eating or "to clean the plate" when they are truly no longer hungry.

Malaria

Globally the malaria situation is serious and worsening with mortality ranging between 1.5-2.7 million and morbidity 300-500 million annually. 90% of the burden is in Africa where it is estimated that it will kill 1 in 20 children under five years of age. 90% of the global burden of disease for malaria is attributable to environmental factors. Malaria affects 40% of the world's population and is most common and severe in pre-school children and pregnant women in Africa.

In school-age children, malaria is estimated to account for between 10-20% of mortality and is an important cause of morbidity. Schoolchildren who have not acquired exposure-driven immunity may be at particularly high risk of severe and fatal consequences when exposed to the disease in unstable transmission areas. Pregnant schoolgirls are also a particular high-risk group. Malaria is also an important cause of absenteeism from school and accounts for between 13-50% of all school days missed because of preventable medical causes.

There is also evidence that brain insult, as a

consequence of cerebral malaria in early childhood, may have an effect on a child's cognitive and learning ability. Like diarrhoea, the priority age group is younger than school age children.

HIV/AIDS

Although human immunodeficiency virus (HIV) and acquired immunodeficiency syndrome (AIDS) and other sexually transmitted diseases (STDs) constitute a relatively modest portion of the burden of disease in school-age children, there is growing evidence that HIV/AIDS constitute a severe threat to the future health and well-being of sexually active school-age children. Population studies in Tanzania have shown that HIV prevalence among adolescents and young adults (15 - 24 years) range from 1% in rural areas to 21% in certain urban areas.

Studies of HIV/AIDS in youth in Uganda estimate that the prevalence of HIV in children aged 13-18 years is relatively low at 2.5% in females and 0.4% in males. These rates increase rapidly, however, to 19.4% in females and 2.7% in males in the 20-24 year age group and amply demonstrate the need to focus HIV/AIDS education programmes at school-age children to reduce the very high risk of mortality associated with HIV-related diseases.

Diarrhoeal diseases

WHO estimates that 3.3 million children die from intestinal infections such as cholera, typhoid or infectious hepatitis every year. The total number of diarrhoeal episodes may be as high as 4000 million. Most of the diarrhoeal disease burden occurs in children in developing countries with under fives at greatest risk. Approximately 90% of the diarrhoeal disease burden is related to environmental factors of poor sanitation and lack of access to clean water and safe food. Where appropriate sanitation facilities and adequate supplies of water for hand-washing and safe water for drinking are either non-existent or inadequate, the school environment can become an added source of disease transmission.

Awareness of Health and Nutrition Programmes

There is a growing awareness and concern for the health and nutrition situation of non-attending school-age children which has prompted an increase in the level of research and programming to identify and address problems in this age group. The evidence from recent studies highlights the importance of early childhood development programmes that prevent stunting in the early years, and the importance of school-based programmes that extend health and nutrition services to out-of-school children.

A failure to extend health and nutrition services to non attending school-age children is likely to exacerbate existing inequalities in society. School enrolment rates vary enormously between regions, within regions and within countries although information on the numbers of non-enrolled children or on those who do not complete their basic education is incomplete.

Delayed enrolment can lead to fewer years in school, poor educational achievement and ultimately poor employment prospects. It is estimated that out of a total 625 million children of primary school age, 79% are in school. Girls' participation in school remains low in many countries, often lagging well behind that of boys. The gender gap for primary school education is particularly high in countries such as Nepal, Pakistan, Benin, Chad and the Yemen.

The factors that limit girls' access to education are varied and include household socio-economic constraints, the demands placed on older girls to nurse sick family members, the onset of menses, teenage pregnancy, early marriage and child labour. A study to examine the relationship between nutritional status and enrolment in primary school children has been carried out in Tanzania and Ghana. It was found that the majority of children enrol late with an average of 1 year late for school-age children in Ghana and 2-3 years late in Tanzania. Delayed school enrolment was found to be significantly associated with short stature in both countries even after controlling for socio-economic status .

There is also a suggestion that the children who are most likely to drop out of school have a worse nutritional status (low height for age) compared with the relatively healthier and taller children who remain in school. Thus the association between short stature and poor enrolment is maintained throughout school. Stunted children, therefore, not only enrol later in school but that are less likely to complete their basic schooling.

In Egypt, a study of school-age children revealed that non-enrolled children had a higher prevalence and infection load of schistosomiasis than enrolled children did. It is calculated that the proportion of infected school-age children who would miss school-based treatment due to non-enrolment could be as high as 60% and that the level of non-inclusion in the control programme is a major factor limiting the programme impact.

There have been numerous studies into the factors that may limit a school child's cognitive development (memory, problem solving, numerical and language skills) and their ability to participate fully in school education. In developing countries, these studies have focussed on the effects of stunting, wasting, micronutrient deficiencies, short-term hunger and more recently, helminth infections. The studies into the effect of undernutrition on cognitive ability although not entirely conclusive do indicate that chronic undernutrition is associated with lower achievement levels in school children.

Impact of School-based nutrition and health programmes

School health and nutrition programmes are the essential sequel and compliment to early child development programs. Good health and nutrition at school age is essential for good education. Freedom from disease promotes intellectual as well as physical development. It enhances school attendance and the ability to learn while at school".

The mass delivery of anthelmintics (deworming medication) and the delivery of micronutrients, particularly iron and iodine are among the most cost-effective, simple and safe school-based programmes that can be delivered by trained teachers. These interventions are only a short-term measure, however, if unaccompanied with appropriate health and nutrition information, education and communication (IEC).

Iron

There have been increased efforts to develop improved interventions for the control of iron deficiency and anaemia involving food fortification, oral supplementation and dietary education as a combined strategy. Adolescent girls are an important target group in iron supplementation programmes in developing countries. This is because their iron requirements are relatively high, they tend to have early pregnancies and supplementation can protect them from iron deficiency during pregnancy that could also benefit foetal development.

Where iron deficiency is a public health problem in school-age children, iron supplementation is recommended even where the costs of purchasing the tablets have to be met by individual family's. Supplementation programmes targeted at pregnant women, however, have been fraught with problems in many developing countries because of weaknesses within health service delivery and because of low compliance with daily tablet intake.

In recent years, a number of studies have suggested that weekly iron supplementation is as effective as daily supplementation in raising haemoglobin levels. Many of these studies have found significant benefits in subjects receiving weekly supplements and there is now a growing momentum for a change in policy from daily to *weekly dosing. However, there is a still a need to further assess the effectiveness of weekly supplements under programme conditions to ensure that compliance is achieved.*

Recent studies from Indonesia and Malaysia have lent weight to these findings and have demonstrated improvements in the iron stores of adolescent schoolgirls supplemented once weekly. In the Indonesian study, the group who received retinol along with the iron supplement benefited most in terms of increased iron stores. The effect of giving micronutrient deficient schoolchildren in South Africa biscuits fortified with iron and with iodine and beta-carotene has been shown to significantly improve their micronutrient status. There is conflicting evidence concerning the beneficial effect of iron supplementation on growth in children. Some studies have shown that daily supplementation improves growth and appetite, while others have not found any beneficial growth response.

Iodine

Universal iodisation of salt is seen as the permanent and sustainable solution to the global IDD problem. Iodisation of salt is the preferred approach for supplementation in iodine deficient populations as its source can be controlled and the technology required is relatively simple. In many countries, it is now mandatory for manufactured salt to be iodised although this does not guarantee the elimination or reduction of IDD. In many countries a persistence of goitre in schoolchildren is being observed despite and apparent successful implementation of near universal iodised salt consumption

In areas where iodised salt is not available and where the prompt correction of IDD is urgent, iodised oil can be administered to schoolchildren relatively cheaply and simply and can maintain iodine levels for a period of twelve months. In Guatemala where the uptake of iodised salt has been problematic, IDD education through schools has been piloted to identify whether the use of school children as health messengers could alter purchasing behaviour at the household level.

In South Africa, where mandatory iodisation of salt was introduced in 1995, a study into the effects on school children in an endemically goitrous area after one year found that iodine deficiency was virtually eradicated in the study population.

Growth of Nutritional Deficit

The intensity of infection, the regularity and duration of treatment and nutritional status have all been identified as important factors that influence programme impact. Overall the growth and nutritional deficits caused by these infections have been shown to be reversible through appropriate treatment. In Guatemala, schoolchildren who were given two treatments for very high levels of Ascaris infection (91%) were found to have modest increases in weight gain 6 months after the initial treatment.

A more recent evaluation study from East Africa into the effect of a school-based deworming programme on growth after one year found that linear growth improved in children who received twice or thrice yearly treatment. Children who were less stunted and who were younger benefited the most although the overall increase in growth did not bring the children in line with the international growth standards.

Helminth infections are prevalent in areas where iron deficiency is widespread. The relationship between hookworm infection and anaemia has been well established in the past and more recent studies show that even light hookworm infections can lead to anaemia in school children when nutritional status is poor. Helminth infection influences iron status through loss of blood, loss of appetite resulting in a reduction in food intake and by interfering with metabolism.

In many schools facilities are either poor or absent and the aim of any school sanitation, hygiene and water programme combine hardware and software. The former revolves around the construction of facilities and their subsequent maintenance and use while the latter focuses on necessary and appropriate learning experiences to encourage safe practice at school, home and throughout later life.

The latter is now referred to as hygiene promotion to distinguish between the former use of didactic teaching of health education and the new approach of participatory growth centred learning. Hygiene promotion is now seen as an intrinsic element of any water and sanitation initiative and, in the context of school health, is now a central focus for the UNICEF school sanitation and hygiene programme.

This approach has the following key elements:

— *the safe, efficient and hygienic disposal of faeces,*

particularly child faeces

— the safe, efficient and hygienic management of water from extraction, through transport and storage to use (particularly for drinking and hand-washing)

— the regular and effective use of water(with a scouring agent like soap or ash) for hand-washing after contact with stools

These three are generally considered to be the most important behavioural domains because they carry the greatest potential risk both on a personal and a communal level. There is increasing recognition of the importance of promoting safe hygiene behaviour among school children not simply because of its importance in the immediate school environment but also because of the communication opportunities and potential influence on the family.

School malaria prevention programmes are a good example of how schools can make a contribution to community health. It is suggested that children can be important agents for change in malaria control programmes. Skills based health education through schools can help promote a community wide understanding of malaria with particular emphasis on the need for community based control measures such as the use of impregnated bed nets.

Schools can serve as a focus for synchronised impregnation of bed nets and distribution. Other types of intervention are less appropriate for the school child as demonstrated in a study from Kenya where the provision through schools of chemoprophylaxis, mass drug administration, selective treatment of infections and fever management with diagnostics were *considered unaffordable options.*

School-based HIV/AIDS education programmes

School-based HIV/AIDS education programmes aim to increase school-age children's knowledge about AIDS, change attitudes toward risk behaviours, delay onset of sexual intercourse and increase condom use among sexually active students. Recent studies indicate that a substantial proportion of primary school children report being sexually active, thus children in primary schools constitute an important target group in AIDS prevention efforts.

In Tanzania the impact of a school-based HIV/AIDS prevention programme has been evaluated one year after implementation. The programme involved training primary school teachers and local health workers for one week in the use of low-cost educational material that they then used for 2-3 months in the classroom. The aim was to increase communication about AIDS, provide information on how students can protect themselves from AIDS and foster restrictive attitudes towards early sexual activity.

It was found that the programme had substantially increased students knowledge of HIV/AIDS and that students were disseminating this information outside the school environment to their parents, other relatives and to religious leaders. It was concluded that it is both feasible and effective to implement culturally specific HIV/AIDS education to primary school children through trained teachers receiving support from local health personnel.

In Uganda, a comprehensive teacher-based AIDS education programme has been piloted in primary and secondary schools based on the WHO/UNESCO School Health Education to Prevent AIDS and STD over a period of one year. Teachers were found to be enthusiastic and willing messengers for AIDS education following adequate training. It was also found that teachers had improved relations with their students as a result of the promotion of open communication methods.

School-based health programmes

School-based health programmes have previously been characterised as being heavily focussed on disease prevention, uncoordinated, lacking integration and poorly evaluated and disseminated. This situation now appears to be improving as those involved in international school health are working more closely together, a move away from individual to multiple strategies is emerging and the dissemination of evidence of effectiveness has increased. There is also the important recognition that schools are, first and foremost, places for learning, and that health and nutrition programmes should neither overload teachers, the curricula or be a burden on schooling.

There are numerous examples of school health and nutrition programmes and approaches. The benefits of an effective school health, hygiene and nutrition programme are likely to include the following:

— *Responds to new need*

— *Increases the efficacy of other investments in child development*

— *Ensures better educational outcomes*

— *Achieves greater social equity*

— *Is highly cost-effective*

School health programmes help link the resources of the health, education, nutrition, and sanitation sectors in an infrastructure - the school—that is already in place, is pervasive and is sustained. While the school system is rarely universal, coverage is often superior to health systems and has an extensive skilled workforce that already works closely with the community. The accessibility of school health programmes to a large proportion of each nation's population, including staff as well as students, contributes to the low cost of programmes.

The high effectiveness of these programmes is a consequence of the synergy between the health benefit and the educational benefit. The effectiveness is measurable in terms not only of improved health and nutrition, but also of improved educational outcomes, reduced wastage, less repetition and generally enhanced returns on educational investments.

School Health and Nutrition Programme

Developing an effective school health component in broader efforts to achieve more child-friendly schools. Much more could be done, but if all schools implement these four interventions then there would be a significant immediate benefit, and a basis for future expansion. In particular, the aim is to focus on interventions that are feasible to implement even in the most resource poor schools, and in hard-to-reach rural areas as well accessible urban areas, that promote learning through improved health and nutrition. Four components that should be made available together, in all schools.

(i) Health-related school policies

Health policies in schools, including skills-based health education and the provision of some health services, can help promote the overall health, hygiene and nutrition of children. But good health policies should go beyond this to ensure a safe and secure physical environment and A positive psycho-social environment, and should address issues such as abuse of students, sexual harassment, school violence, and bullying. By guaranteeing the further education of pregnant schoolgirls and young mothers, school health policies will help promote inclusion and equity in the school environment.

Policies that help to prevent and reduce harassment by other students and even by teachers, also help to fight against reasons that girls withdraw or are withdrawn from schools. Policies regarding the health-related practices of teachers and students can reinforce health education: teachers can act as positive role models for their students, for example, by not smoking in school. The process of developing and agreeing upon policies draws attention to these issues. The policies are best developed by involving many levels, including the national level, and teachers, children, and parents at the *school level.*

(ii) Provision of safe water and sanitation - the essential first steps towards a healthy physical, learning environment.

The school environment may damage the health and nutritional status of schoolchildren, particularly if it increases their exposure to hazards such as infectious disease carried by the water supply. Hygiene education is meaningless without clean water and adequate sanitation facilities. It is a realistic goal in most countries to ensure that all schools have access to clean water and sanitation.

By providing these facilities, schools can reinforce the health and hygiene messages, and act as an example to both students and the wider community. This in turn can lead to a demand for similar facilities from the community. Sound construction policies will help ensure that facilities address issues such as gender access and privacy. Separate facilities for girls, particularly adolescent girls, are an important contributing factor to reducing dropout at menses and even before. Sound maintenance policies will help ensure the continuing safe use of these facilities.

(iii) Skills based health education

This approach to health, hygiene and nutrition education focuses upon the development of knowledge, attitudes, values, and life skills needed to make and act on the most appropriate and positive health-related decisions. Health in this context extends beyond physical health to include psycho-social and environmental health issues.

Changes in social and behavioural factors have given greater prominence to such health- related issues as HIV/AIDS, early pregnancy, injuries, violence and tobacco and substance use. Unhealthy social and behavioural factors not only influence lifestyles, health and nutrition, but also hinder education opportunities for a growing number of school-age children and adolescents.

The development of attitudes related to gender equity and respect between girls and boys, and the development of specific skills, such as dealing with peer pressure, are central to effective skills based health education and positive psycho-social environments. When individuals have such skills they are more likely to adopt and sustain a healthy lifestyle during schooling and for the rest of their lives.

(iv) School based health and nutrition services

Schools can effectively deliver some health and nutritional services provided that the services are simple, safe and familiar, and address problems that are prevalent and recognized as important within the community. If these criteria are met then the community sees the teacher and school more positively, and teachers perceive themselves as playing important roles. For example, micronutrient deficiencies and worm infections may be effectively dealt with by infrequent (six-monthly or annual) oral treatment; changing the timing of meals, or providing a snack to address short term hunger during school - an important constraint on learning - can contribute to school performance; and providing spectacles will allow some children to fully participate in class for the first time.

v Supporting Activities

These activities provide the context in which the interventions can be implemented.

(i) *Effective partnerships between teachers and health workers and between the education and health sectors : The success of school health programmes demands an effective partnership between Ministries of Education and Health, and between teachers and health workers. The health sector retains the responsibility for the health of children, but the education sector is responsible for implementing, and often funding, the school based programmes. These sectors need to identify responsibilities and present a coordinated action to improve health and learning outcomes from children.*

(ii) *Effective community partnerships: Promoting a positive interaction between the school and the community is fundamental to the success and sustainability of any school improvement process. Community partnerships engender a sense of collaboration, commitment and communal ownership. Such partnerships also build public awareness and strengthen demand. Within the school health component of such improvement processes, parental support and cooperation allows education about* health to be shared and reinforced at home. The involvement of the broader community (the private sector, community organizations and women's groups) can enhance and reinforces school health promotion and resources. These partnerships, which should work together to make schools more child-friendly, can jointly identify health issues that need to be addressed through the school and then help design and manage activities to address such issues.

(iii) *Pupil awareness and participation:* Children must be important participants in all aspects of school health programmes, and not simply the beneficiaries. Children who participate in: health policy development and implementation; efforts to create a safer and more sanitary environment; health promotion aimed at their parents, other children, and community members; and school health services, learn about health by doing. This is an effective way to help young people acquire the knowledge, attitudes, values and skills needed to adopt healthy lifestyles and to support health and Education for All.

Ensuring that children are healthy and able to learn is an essential component of an effective education system. Good health increases enrollment and reduces absenteeism, and brings more of the poorest and most disadvantaged children to school, many of whom are girls. It is these children who are often the least healthy and most malnourished, and who have the most to gain educationally from improved health.

Effective school health programs that are developed as part of community partnerships provide one of the most cost-effective ways to reach school age children, *adolescents and the broader community, and are a sustainable way to promote healthy practices including HIV/AIDS prevention.*

The new FRESH framework (Focusing Resources on Effective School Health) is the starting point for developing an effective school health, hygiene and nutrition program in a more child friendly and health promoting school. An effective school health, hygiene and nutrition program such as FRESH offers many benefits:

It responds to an increased need

The success of child survival programs and the efforts of many governments and communities to expand basic education coverage have resulted both in a greater number of school-age children and in a greater proportion of these children attending school. Almost 90% of the world's children survive beyond their fifth birthday and some 80% of these children are enrolled in school. In many countries, targeted education programs have ensured that many of these new entrants are girls for whom good health is especially important. Additionally, school aged children are the window of hope in the fight against HIV/AIDS. HIV/AIDS prevention is needed in schools.

It increases the efficacy of other investments in child development

School health programs are the essential sequel and complement to early child care and development programs. Continuing good health at school age is essential if children are to sustain the advantages of a healthy early childhood and take full advantage of what may be their only opportunity for formal learning.

Ensures better educational outcomes

Ensuring good health at school-age can boost school enrollment and attendance, reduce the need for repetition, and increase educational attainment. Good health practices can promote reproductive health and help avoid HIV/AIDS. It is estimated that the burden of disease for school-aged children 5-14 years is 11% of the total global burden of disease.

It improves social equity

As a result of universal basic education strategies, some of the most disadvantaged children - girls, poor rural children, children with disabilities - have access to school for the first time. But their ability to attend school and to learn whilst there is compromised by poor health. These are the children who will benefit most from health interventions, since they are likely to show the greatest improvements in attendance and learning achievement.

It is a highly cost effective strategy

School health programs help link resources for health, education, nutrition, and sanitation to an infrastructure the school - that is already in place, is pervasive and is sustained. While the school system is rarely universal, coverage is often superior to health systems. And the school system has an extensive skilled workforce that already works closely with the community.

The FRESH framework for School Health interventions includes health-related school policies, provision of water and sanitation, skills-based health education and health and nutrition services in schools. The FRESH framework was developed by a partnership of UNESCO, UNICEF, WHO and the World Bank, and launched at the World Education Forum, April 2000.

The framework is the starting point for developing an effective school health hygiene and nutrition program in a more child friendly and health promoting school. The aim is to focus on interventions that are feasible to implement even in the most resource-poor schools. The core framework has four components that should be made available in all schools:

1. *Health-related school policies that, for example, do not exclude pregnant girls, that encourage healthy tobacco-free lifestyles, and that help maintain the education system in the face of HIV/AIDS.*
2. *Access to safe water and provision of sanitation to provide a healthy learning environment that reinforces hygienic behaviors and provides privacy to promote participation of adolescent girls in education.*
3. *Skills-based approach to health, hygiene, and nutrition education that focuses upon the development of knowledge, attitudes, values, and life skills needed to establish lifelong healthy practices and to reduce the vulnerability of youth and teachers to HIV/AIDS.*
4. *School-based health and nutrition services that are simple, safe and familiar, and address problems that are prevalent and recognized as important within the community, including the provision of counseling to cope with the HIV/AIDS epidemic.*

3

Health Promotion

Oral Health

Oral health enables an individual to speak, eat and socialise without active disease, discomfort or embarrassment. Oral health is fundamental to general health and well being, significantly impacting on quality of life. It can affect general health conditions. Oral health means more than healthy teeth. The health of the gums, oral soft tissues, chewing muscles, the palate, tongue, lips and salivary glands are also significant.

Poor oral health can have a detrimental effect on children's performance in school and their success in later life. Children who suffer from poor oral health are 12 times more likely to have more restricted-activity days including missing school than those who do not. More than 50 million hours annually are lost from school due to oral diseases.

While tooth decay (dental caries) and gum disease (inflammatory periodontal disease) are among the most prevalent or widespread conditions in human populations, other conditions such as trauma of teeth and jaws, dental erosion, developmental enamel defects and oral cancer are also important. Premature loss of deciduous (milk) teeth may lead to malalignment of the permanent (adult) teeth, impacting on an individual's appearance.

Importantly, tooth loss can affect children's nutritional intake and, consequently, their growth and development. Poor oral hygiene causes gum disease and, together with dietary sugars, dental decay. Both conditions may lead to pain, discomfort and tooth loss. Tooth loss, as a result of untreated dental disease and trauma, may have a profound impact on quality of life, as well as on growth and development.

While there has been improvement in oral health of children in the last few decades, tooth decay remains one of the most common childhood diseases, in both industrialised and developing countries. A substantial proportion of children in many developing countries are affected by tooth decay, and most decay is left untreated due to limited access to oral health services.

The occurrence of gum disease is high among older children and adolescents, with 50% to 100% of 12-years-old children having the signs of gum inflammation. It is almost omnipresent among adults. Dental trauma, which usually affects the upper front teeth, may result from accidents, sport-related injuries, violence, and epilepsy. Traumatised baby teeth may lead to tooth loss and, among other factors such as childhood illnesses, may affect the developing permanent teeth.

It is therefore important to prevent dental trauma

in children. A safe environment at home, in schools and in the community, including safer playgrounds and roads with well-organised traffic, can help minimise the risks. Dental erosion, a form of tooth wear that is linked to increased consumption of carbonated and fruit drinks, is becoming a problem in some countries, although occasionally it may be due to repeated vomiting.

In most cases, abnormal tooth wear results in a loss of normal enamel contour, but in severe cases the interior of the tooth may be affected. Other forms of tooth wear, attrition and abrasion, are related to tooth grinding habits, and abrasive dietary and inappropriate oral hygiene practices (e.g. brushing with a hard brush, abrasive toothpaste or other materials such as powder and charcoal).

Oral cancer is on the increase, becoming the 11 th most common cancer in the world, with a 5-year survival rate of less than 50%. The prevalence of oral cancer varies greatly between countries, with a particularly high incidence observed in the Indian subcontinent, Australia, France, South America and Sub-Saharan Africa. While 95% of the disease cases are diagnosed among adults aged over 40 years, risk behaviours during childhood and adolescence could have a significant impact on the risk of cancer, as well as other leading cause of death and disability.

Cigarette smoking and "spit or chewing" tobacco use among adolescents in the US has been increasing each year, with 35% of those who use tobacco having tobacco-related oral lesions. Other tobacco containing products that are marketed directly at children and adolescents include pan masala, bidis and ghutka. With attractive packaging and flavours, they are often mistaken as sweets.

The school years cover a period that runs from childhood to adolescence. These are influential stages in people's lives when lifelong sustainable oral health related behaviours, as well as beliefs and attitudes, are being developed. Children are particularly receptive during this period and the earlier the habits are established, the longer lasting the impact. Moreover, the messages can be reinforced regularly throughout the school years.

Children may also be equipped with personal skills that enable them to make healthy decisions, to adopt a healthy lifestyle and to deal with stressful situations such as violence and conflicts. Schools can provide a supportive environment for promoting oral health. For example, the provision of safe water and sanitation facilities is essential for toothbrushing activities in schools. The school does not have such facilities, oral health promotion can trigger the installation of these basic facilities.

A safe physical environment in the playgrounds, and indeed throughout the school, can help reduce the risk of dental trauma. With the appropriate policies and practices, vital actions can be taken in case of emergency. Such actions can save the traumatised tooth/teeth, avoiding tooth loss and associated problems in later life. School policies and practices on healthy diet that ensure healthy foods and drinks are provided in all areas, particularly policies on sugar intake, serve to promote healthy dietary behaviours from an early age.

More importantly, schools may be the only place

for children, who are at the highest risk of dental disease, to have access to oral health services. This is particularly true in many developing countries, compounded by a lack of dental personnel. With adequate training, school teachers can play an important role in oral health activities.

Schools can also provide an important network and channel to the local community. Health promotion activities can be targeted at the home and throughout the community by school personnel. Similarly, through the pupils, health promotion messages can be passed on to other members of the family. Schools can also take the lead role in advocating and lobbying for general as well as oral health. This school-home-community interaction is an important aspect a Health-Promoting School.

While there have been improvements in dental health over the past decades and many children today enjoy good oral health, many do not. There is not a single country that claims to be 'caries free'. Tooth decay is one of the most common chronic childhood diseases. For example, in the US it is 5 times more common than asthma and 7 times more common than hay fever.

In the Philippines, it has been reported that dental decay outranks the combined rates of other diseases in the country. In the WHO South-East Asia and Eastern Mediterranean regions, dental decay is an important cause of disability. There are variations across countries, and disparities between regions, provinces, districts, cities and areas. While there has been a significant decline in tooth decay in some developed countries during the past few decades, a large number of children worldwide are still suffering from the disease, much of *which is active and untreated, leading to toothache and restricted activities.*

Such problems are particularly prevalent among children of deprived communities. Similar to tooth decay, gum disease affects children in all countries and, in many countries, it is one of the most common diseases. The prevalence of gum disease in children is very high worldwide, with the majority of children being affected.

Unintentional injury is one of the leading causes of death in the world, with 1 in 5 deaths among children under the age of 15 years. In some developing countries, unintentional injuries account for 80% of all deaths in children. Sport and playground related injuries, as well as general and road traffic accidents, often affect the head, neck and mouth. These injuries have a significant impact on oral health.

Throughout the world, the number of cases of head and face injuries is increasing in both urban and rural areas. With the increase in road traffic, poor lighting on the road and a lack of legislation regarding road safety, this is particularly significant in some developing countries. The front teeth are most vulnerable.

In some countries, over 50% of children have experienced oral trauma, with a quarter of cases being children under the age of 5 years. According to the 1993 UK Child Dental Health Survey, 5% of 12-year-old children exhibit trauma to their front teeth. The corresponding figure for Syria is 12%. In the US, over 20% of children aged less than 15 years have been admitted to the emergency room sustaining head and face injuries. While the most commonly sustained damage is fractures to tooth enamel, some injuries can lead to permanent tooth loss.

The significance of intentional head and face injuries should not be overlooked. In addition to potential direct damage to the teeth and, possibly, other head and face structures, they may be signs of child abuse, a problem that could scar the child for life.

Defects and the colour of tooth enamel affect the appearance of teeth which, in turn, may have a impact on quality of life. The prevalence of enamel undesirable and defects is rising in some countries. Demarcated opacities (white marks on the teeth) are often found on the upper front teeth, while diffuse opacities or fluorosis (discolouration of the teeth) affect all the teeth generally.

Some childhood systemic diseases and malnutrition during tooth formation could lead to hypoplasia (discolouration and structural damage to the teeth). In some countries, about 25-40% of children have opacities (demarcated or diffuse opacities) of the tooth enamel on one or more teeth. In Malaysia, it has been reported that over 75% of 12-year-old children have some form of enamel defects and opacities, regardless of whether the area is fluoridated or not. However, severe enamel defects are not common.

Many children, their parents and teachers have inadequate oral health knowledge and awareness. In many countries, a considerable number of children have limited knowledge of the causes and prevention of the most common oral disease. Similarly, mothers' oral health knowledge is generally poor and schoolteachers' oral health knowledge, while better than that of the mothers', remains unsatisfactory.

It is evident that cultural beliefs play an important role in the perception of the causes of dental decay and *gum disease. Only a small proportion of children, parents and schoolteachers is aware of the harmful effects of hidden sugars and sugary drinks. Moreover, while many parents recognise the importance of toothbrushing in general, some do not know how to prevent tooth decay and gum disease and the role of fluoride in the prevention of dental decay is poorly understood.*

In many countries, less than half of mothers have received oral health advice from dentists. While the harmful effect of smoking is generally acknowledged, other forms of tobacco use are not regarded as risk factors for oral cancer. Many children are exposed to smoke because their parents smoke at home. Improving the parents' awareness, attitudes and behaviour toward tobacco is therefore paramount.

Many children are not adopting practices that are essential to maintain good oral health As part of oral hygiene routine self-care, children should clean their teeth and gums every day with fluoridated toothpaste. However, in many countries the proportion of children who brush their teeth every day is still unsatisfactory.

A small proportion of children does not clean their teeth at all. Some may not have access to a toothbrush. The use of traditional cleaning aids such as 'Miswaki', a traditional chewing stick, is common in some communities. Furthermore, the availability, affordability and quality of fluoride toothpaste remain a major problem in developing countries. Only a small proportion of children used fluoridated toothpaste.

In some countries, toothpastes are considered as cosmetics with high taxation, leading to exorbitant retail prices that are out of reach of most families. The need for promoting affordable fluoride toothpaste is evident. In several countries, many households do not have access to safe water for drinking, let alone for cleaning teeth. Given that schools may be the only place where children can carry out oral hygiene practices, it is therefore vital that sufficient safe water and sanitation facilities are provided in schools.

Healthy dietary behaviours are essential to growth and development and to maintain good oral health. The relationship between diet and oral disease is well established. It is therefore essential to reduce the amount, and more importantly the frequency, of sugary foods, snacks and drinks in a well-balanced diet with sufficient fresh fruit and vegetables. However, a high proportion of schoolchildren aged 11 to 17 years consume sugary snacks daily, according to a recent international report on health behaviour in schoolchildren.

In many countries, over 50% of 15-year-old children drink at least one can of soft drink everyday. In order to reduce the risk of oral cancer in later life, it is important to start at a very young age to have a balanced and healthy diet, to avoid using tobacco and consuming alcohol, to limit the exposure to the sun and to protect the lips from overexposure. Addressing these risk factors also helps prevent other oral diseases and general health conditions.

However, in many countries, children and adolescents are increasingly developing a habit of tobacco use, in the form of cigarette smoking or smokeless tobacco. In Greenland, over 50% of 15-year-old children smoke daily and 3 in 4 smokers in the region of the Americas start smoking during adolescence. Over 50% of children as young as 8 years old have experienced chewing tobacco in some communities. In some cultures, children chew betel quid that contains tobacco and other carcinogens. The high sugar content in some chewing tobacco is also a cause for concern.

Professional care is an important component for attaining and maintaining optimal oral health. However, a significant proportion of children have no access to dental care, particularly among children in developing countries. A staggering number of children have not visited a dentist before starting school. In some countries, a significant proportion of school children has never visited the dentist. For example, in Tanzania, over 75% of 12- year-old children have never been to the dentist.

Consequently, few have preventive oral care. Many children go to see the dentist when in pain, an experience that may have a lasting effect through life and prove to be detrimental to oral health. Most advanced oral diseases are irreversible. For example, once tooth decay in permanent teeth is established, it will last for a lifetime. Even when the decayed teeth have been restored, the fillings remain in the mouth for life and may need to be replaced from time to time.

However, it must be emphasised that, with appropriate measures, early onset of gum disease and dental decay is reversible. In contrast, advanced or established lesions progressively become more serious and difficult to treat. Clearly, prevention is better than cure.

The oral health of children is a significant public

health issue. Oral disease is one of the most costly diet- and behaviour-related diseases. Childhood oral diseases, if untreated, can lead to irreversible damage, pain, disfigurement, more serious general health problems, lost school time, low self-esteem, poor quality of life and, in the case of noma, death. The delay in treatment not only results in aggravation of disease, but also costs of care are substantially escalated as a consequence.

Adverse dental experience during childhood may lead to dental phobia, impacting on attitudes to oral health and self-care as well as dental visiting behaviours for life. These could have further personal and treatment costs. Oral diseases result in considerable costs. Dental services constitute about 5% to 10% of the total health expenditure in industrial countries each year, costing billions of dollars.

This poses a problem to many developing countries. The cost of dental treatment could easily exhaust the country's entire health budget, a budget that is already fully stretched or simply does not exist. The social and educational costs are also significant. For example, over 50 million school hours in learning are lost due to dental problems in the US. The interference with daily activities, sleeping pattern, quality of life and parents' work output is considerable.

Prevention, early diagnosis and timely treatment are therefore crucial in efforts to contain the costs of oral diseases. Children with disabilities are at increased risk of oral diseases, infections, delayed tooth eruption, gum disease and enamel defects. The exposure to special diets, medications and therapies, compounded by difficulty in maintaining effective self-care practices and in accessing professional care, have a serious adverse *effect on their oral health.*

Costs of neglect are also high, in terms of financial, social and personal impacts. Advanced disease may necessitate more complex, costly and, possibly, more traumatic treatments, such as surgery, root canal therapy, extractions and treatment under general anaesthesia and hospitalisation. Playground related injuries, including injuries to head and face, among children aged 15 years or under cost the US government an estimated 1.2 billion dollars annually.

There are also indirect and intangible costs that should not be underestimated. Poor oral health in childhood often continues into adulthood, impacting on economic productivity and quality of life. It has been reported that investment in oral disease prevention and health promotion decreases costs in health expenditure and is more cost-effective in the long-term.

Poor oral health affects learning, general health and well being. The experience of pain, endurance of dental abscesses, problems with eating and chewing, embarrassment about the discoloration, damage or shape of teeth can distract children from play and effective learning. Oral health affects general health. If left untreated even for a short period of time, oral diseases can have adverse consequences.

Oral infection can kill. It has been considered a risk factor for a number of general health conditions. Systemic spread of germs can cause, or seriously worsen, infections throughout the body, particularly among individuals with suppressed immune systems, heart disease and diabetes.

Studies have suggested that oral diseases (such as

dental decay and gum disease) are associated with a variety of problems. For example:

- *failure to thrive;*
- *poor nutrition;*
- *speech impairments;*
- *psychological problems;*
- *cardiovascular disease;*
- *diabetes;*
- *cancer.*

Furthermore, some common medications and therapies used to treat general health conditions can compromise the health of the mouth and oral functioning. In recent years, much research has demonstrated the impact of oral health on quality of life. A number of oral health related quality of life measures have been developed to assess the functional, psychological, social and economic consequences.

In general, poor oral health has a negative impact on quality of life, influencing eating abilities, personal confidence, mental health, social interaction, personal relationships, general health and well being and enjoyment in life. Low quality of life scores are also related to poor oral health status and reduced access to professional care. Similarly, general health risk factors also affect oral health, such as excessive alcohol intake, smoking, tobacco use and poor dietary practices.

The correlation between these lifestyle behaviours and increased risk of tooth decay, gum disease, oral infections, head and face defects, oral cancer and other oral conditions has been evidenced. There is a need to adopt an integrated approach to address these important risk factors for both oral and general health. Promoting oral health provides a valuable opportunity to integrate oral health promotion into general health promotion.

Such an approach is likely to be more efficient and effective than those programmes targeting a single disease or condition. Poor oral health affects the growth, development and well being of children and has a significant impact on later life. Nutrition plays a critical role in a number of oral diseases including dental decay, gum disease, toothwear and oral cancer.

Nutrition and oral health have a particularly intricate relationship. They form a vicious circle; poor oral health disrupts nutritional intake and poor nutrition affects the development of oral tissues including teeth, making them more susceptible to oral disease. Chronic deficiencies of some micronutrients, such as ascorbate, zinc and iron, may also impair the oral defence mechanisms. Poor oral health is associated with stunted growth and compromised nutrition.

Early childhood caries (ECC) could lead to failure to thrive. ECC has been considered an indicator for malnutrition, a condition that affects growth and development of children. Mental development and, subsequently, learning abilities are compromised. In more severe cases, malnutrition can cause death. Nutritional deficiencies could also lead to many general health problems in later life such as cardiovascular diseases and poor pregnancy outcomes.

In contrast, good oral health helps promote nutritional intake in children, enhancing their learning potential and school performance and enabling them to lead a more productive life. Many oral conditions, diseases or disorders are preventable through school-based efforts. Effective oral hygiene practices, good dietary behaviours and appropriate use of fluorides, together with sustainable, effective and accessible professional care, are keys to good oral health.

The school provides an excellent setting for delivering oral health services for children. Individuals, families, community, schools, education authorities, healthcare providers and government departments should work collaboratively to reduce risk factors and to promote oral health, incorporating the guiding principles for health promotion:

— *develop healthy public policies;*

— *create supportive environments;*

— *strengthen community actions,*

— *develop personal skills to improve knowledge, attitudes and behaviours;*

— *reorient health services to provide a sustainable, effective and accessible system.*

Healthy behaviours and lifestyles developed at a young age are more sustainable. Prevention is a critically important strategy for promoting good oral health among young people. Most risk behaviours and lifestyles stem from school-age years. Equally, good habits that are developed at a young age are more sustainable. Oral hygiene practices can easily be adopted and incorporated into daily routines such as eating and cooking. Hence, daily toothbrushing with fluoridated toothpaste is a habit that should be encouraged to become a norm early in life.

Good dietary patterns should also be fostered at a young age, particularly in preventing children from acquiring a 'sweet tooth' that leads to a habit of eating too much sugar. Early dental visiting experience enables children to develop a good rapport and relationship with the dental team, so that preventive measures can be implemented before oral disease begins. Parents also play an important role in shaping the positive attitudes and influencing good oral health behaviours at home.

With regular reinforcement and encouragement at home and in schools, these healthy behaviours are more likely to continue into adulthood, becoming life-long habits. Oral health promotion can be integrated into general health promotion and into school curriculum and activities. Oral health promotion activities can easily be integrated into school curriculum and activities, co-ordinated and delivered by school teachers or other school personnel.

In Thailand, school teachers are responsible for oral health education, supervising toothbrushing drills after lunch and oral health screening and surveillance. Many of these activities are also incorporated into general health promotion. For example, oral hygiene forms part of the personal hygiene and grooming programmes such as hair and hand washing. Dental trauma prevention is included in injury prevention.

Oral health surveillance is an integral part of growth and nutrition surveillance that takes place twice a year. Some schools also include oral health in family planning and sex education. Oral health can also be featured in various grade levels throughout the school curriculum, with community projects and home-based activities that involve other members of the family. Oral health-related topics and issues can be introduced in subjects such as science, chemistry, biology, language, arithmetic, social studies, arts and music.

Other general health promotion activities also have oral health significance such as healthy eating. School policies and practices that promote good nutrition, healthy behaviours and self-esteem, and discourage smoking, tobacco use, alcohol consumption and substance abuse are also relevant to oral health. Undoubtedly, the co-operation from schools and teachers is crucial to the development of an effective oral health promotion effort.

School is an efficient setting for oral health promotion. Schools are microcosms of the larger community. With existing structures and systems in place, schools provide excellent opportunities for integrating oral health into the curriculum that is acceptable, appropriate and effective. Children are receptive to guidance and they are familiar with the learning environment and culture in school.

Schools can effectively inform and influence students' oral health knowledge, beliefs, attitudes and behaviour. It is important to target children, particularly at kindergartens and primary schools. Pupils need to acquire knowledge and skills that facilitate a healthy lifestyle and help them cope with social and peer pressure.

Children are empowered to take control over their own health early in their lives and are encouraged to develop positive attitudes toward preventive measures. This is particularly crucial when they reach adolescence when they are challenged and exposed to risk factors such as tobacco and alcohol use and poor dietary practices.

They become more mobile and travel independently in motor vehicles and bicycles, and engage more in sports and other high-risk activities that are more prone to craniofacial injuries. They may begin to experiment with sexual practices during this period, potentially subjecting themselves to infections that predispose to general and oral health problems.

School policies and physical environment are also imperative in the attainment of optimal health. Policies on diet, particularly in relation to sugars and carbonated drinks, are necessary to enable the canteen and tuck shops to promote healthy eating and sensible sugar intake. Many schools in Asia have implemented a daily supervised toothbrushing drill at lunchtime policy, according to a recent report.

A safe physical environment in schools, particularly in play areas, helps reduce craniofacial injuries. With appropriate dental trauma policies in place, timely actions can be taken in case of emergency to minimise permanent damage. Policies on bullying and violence between students, supported by education and empowerment, also help prevent intentional injuries. The provision of safe water and sanitation, together with pollution free environments, is a prerequisite for health.

While access to safe water and sanitation facilities is a human right, about 1.1 billion people in the world have no access to safe drinking water and 2.4 billion lack basic sanitation facilities, most notably in Asian and African countries. Without such facilities, health education and promotion are futile. More importantly, *the school environment may be hazardous to children's health and well being.*

In contrast, by providing these facilities, schools are able to promote effective learning, to reinforce health messages and, particularly for oral health, to undertake health promotion activities. Schools, a well-established system, have the potential to reach a large group of people efficiently.

Schools are more widely distributed even in rural areas of developing countries than health centres and clinics. This is particularly relevant to community-based preventive programmes for dental decay such as milk and water fluoridation schemes. On the other hand, special attention can be given to students who are more susceptible to, or at a higher risk of, oral disease. Working collaboratively with the health services, dental treatment and preventive oral health measures can be made available in the school, a cost-effective approach with minimum disruption to learning and school activities.

Children are encouraged to develop a good relationship with the dental team and a positive attitude towards regular dental attendance. The school dental clinic also provides important physical facilities for baseline assessment, monitoring, research and evaluation. Furthermore, schools are often seen as a place for oral health knowledge and information by parents and the local community.

This lay referral system for obtaining information is common in many countries and teachers play an important role in this process. It is therefore imperative that teachers and school staff are equipped with adequate oral health knowledge and skills. Schools form the heart of the community, a means for social networking for parents through local events and meetings. The schools can capitalise this school-home-community interaction to address common concerns, to form a united force to lobby for water fluoridation and healthy environments in the community where they live, work and learn.

School-based oral health promotion programmes are effective School environments have a significant impact on sustainable healthy behaviours, a key success factor for Health-Promoting Schools. Initiatives that target improving environments in schools for children are largely cost-effective. However, without supportive environments, optimal oral health for children cannot be realised.

There is considerable evidence to support the effectiveness of well-conducted school-based oral health promotion interventions worldwide. In the region of the Americas, the US Surgeon General Report documents that most school-based or community-wide oral health preventive interventions are beneficial and cost-effective.

Most school-based or school-linked fluoride and fissure sealant programmes are effective, particularly for children with high risk of dental decay. Tobacco use prevention and control programmes, as part of the school curriculum, are highly effective in influencing behaviour change. Along with the community-based and media-based activities, school-based programmes are effective in preventing or delaying smoking onset in 20% to 40% of adolescents.

Schools that adopt and implement the principles of a Health-Promoting School ('supportive schools') have a lower proportion of children with tooth decay and dental trauma, compared with 'non-supportive schools'; the more comprehensive the curriculum, the better the oral health outcomes and less inequalities in oral health within the school. In the European region, a comprehensive school-based oral health promotion programme has been in place for decades in some countries.

Working closely with schools, the Danish Municipal Dental Health Service provides comprehensive oral health care to children and adolescents in school, with strong emphasis on prevention and health education to students, school staff and parents. Long-term epidemiological data show that dental knowledge, attitudes and behaviour have improved over time, as has children's oral health status. Wi t h improved dental knowledge and attitudes, parents are more involved in caring for their children's oral health.

There are a number of school-based oral health promotion initiatives undertaken in Ireland, including the Mighty Mouth programme, Den TV and, while not exclusively about oral health, the Nutrition Education At Primary School and Social Personal and Health Education programmes. The programmes adopt the ethos of a Health-Promoting School and show promise. Children's oral health related knowledge, attitudes and behaviour, most notably healthy food choices, have improved.

In Central and Eastern Europe, school oral health programmes were established but brought to a halt during health systems transition. The effect of a school-based oral health promotion programme is more apparent in Hungary. A nation-wide programme was *introduced in 1986 but ceased to exist in the mid-1990s during the health care reform. The oral health of children has improved after the introduction of the programme but deteriorated since the programme has stopped, according to national studies carried out in 1985, 1991 and 1996.*

In the Western Pacific region, an oral health education programme has been undertaken in Wuhan, China, based on the concept of Health-Promoting Schools with a special emphasis on healthy environments and capacity building. A study in Indonesia investigates the long-term effect of a school-based oral health education programme. While there is a significantly better oral health knowledge in the test group, toothbrushing behaviour, oral hygiene status and other oral health behaviours are found to be similar to those of the control group.

An oral health promotion effectiveness review in Australia shows that the use of a settings approach in promoting oral health can potentially lead to oral health benefits, with Health-Promoting Schools being most promising. The importance of supportive school environments is emphasised. A number of studies with this approach have proved to be effective. Evidence suggests that interventions that are incorporated into school curricula, part of other health promotion activities and needs-driven are most successful.

Programmes targeting parents, preschool children, schoolchildren and adolescents have made an impact on knowledge, healthy behaviour and, in some cases, health gains. Similar findings have been reported in New Zealand. Well-designed school-based initiatives that aim at improving knowledge and social competence are generally effective.

In addition, the school dental service is a valuable means of promoting health and equity. In Cambodia, oral health promotion activities form part of the school curriculum, including general and oral health education, daily toothbrushing drills and a weekly fluoride rinse programme. Some activities are led by student leaders, supervised by teachers.

As a result of the programme, significant improvements in oral health knowledge and good practices among children have been reported, particularly in those schools that are more co-operative. In India, oral health education has been integrated into the school curriculum, aiming to provide dental knowledge and to empower children to take control over their own health. Oral health is featured in other subjects, including language, arts, arithmetic, sciences, social studies and music.

Compared with the control groups, the test groups showed a significant improvement in knowledge and oral hygiene. In the African region, oral Health Promoting Schools have been implemented in Madagascar. The initiative has been shown to be effective in improving dental health status and in influencing oral health knowledge and behaviour, compared with the control group. Parents are very supportive of the programme. Consequently, the levels of family support in oral care have also increased.

In South Africa, a 7-year school-based preventive programme results in a significantly lower prevalence and experience of tooth decay, compared with those who did not receive the programme. Similarly, in the region of the Eastern Mediterranean, a 9-year school-based oral health programme in Kuwait also shows an improvement in oral health in children. The programme includes bi-weekly supervised toothbrushing with fluoridated toothpaste and regular fluoride mouthrinse, fissure sealant and restorative dental treatment provided in schools, oral health education delivered by teachers and regularly oral health education programmes for parents and teachers.

Interventions that adopt the Health-Promoting School approach are generally successful. Effectiveness of school health education is associated with the amount of classroom or curricular time devoted to the programme, the extent to which the programme is supported and the commitment of teachers and students. However, the concept and application of a Health-promotion School, or even health promotion, may not be well understood by dental service providers.

In order to fully integrate oral health promotion activities in the school curriculum, training and professional development for teachers are imperative. A comprehensive programme of professional development for teachers improves their skills in, and commitment to, sustaining oral health promotion innovations. Strategies that fit in with wider school and community initiatives are more sustainable. Working in partnership with parents and the local community enhances health gain and the impact of the programmes.

While not all school-based programmes have encompassed all the components of a Health-Promoting School, it is encouraging that some schools have already made a sterling effort in incorporating oral health promotion activities in the school curriculum. It is necessary to build on the good work and achievements, broadening the efforts to maximise the full potential of a Health-Promoting School.

Integrated school-based oral health promotion programmes are cost effective, leading to sustainable cost savings. The cost-effectiveness of school-based programmes in enhancing the health and development of school-age children has been well established. The cost-effectiveness ratios are likely to improve when employing an integrated approach that addresses a number of health and educational problems.

While the true benefits of school-based health promotion interventions may be difficult to ascertain in money terms, they have significant potential for cost savings. In general, the cost per capita of community preventive programmes is lower than that of treatment services. A multifaceted school oral health programme, complemented by water fluoridation, has led to a significant improvement in dental health, with a substantial cost savings.

The proportion of children with no experience of dental decay has increased from 0% to 34%. In countries without fluoridated water, school-based oral health programmes, combined with the use of fluoridated toothpaste, are also cost-effective. Since the implementation of the nationwide school oral health programme, the oral hygiene and oral health of schoolchildren have improved, leading to a significant saving of 3.5 million US dollars.

School-based oral health promotion intervention can benefit the entire community. Oral health promotion can trigger the installation of safe water supply and sanitation facilities in schools; this in turn may lead to a demand for similar facilities from the community. Parents and community members who are involved in the Health-Promoting School Initiative are aware of the important benefits of these facilities.

The training and experience gained in working with others and in gathering resources can prove invaluable in lobbying for better environments at home and in the community. The school, parents and community members can support each other in the process. Children have an important role to play in oral health promotion. Health-Promoting Schools empower children to take control over their health and become an active and responsible citizen in society.

They are encouraged to impart their knowledge to benefit other members of the family and society. This 'spread of effect' of oral health promotion has been documented. Children may have a strong influence on their family and community. Teachers are very supportive of the initiatives. According to the results of a number of surveys, teachers are willing to teach oral health education as part of their routine school activities. Teachers are acutely aware of the poor oral health conditions of their pupils and are willing to take a more active role in oral health promotion in schools.

Some, for example in Thailand, consider it is their duty to help children maintain good oral health. In Tanzania, teachers in primary schools integrate oral health promotion activities in the school curriculum. However, schoolteachers may not have the necessary oral health knowledge and skills to carry out oral health promotion tasks effectively. Many would like to have more training in this area. Consequently, some are reluctant to teach oral health.

In contrast, teachers in many other countries feel strongly about children's oral health and are happy to play a part in oral health education. The willingness of schoolteachers in this role is evident. Oral health can be an effective entry point for building a school's capacity to plan and implement a wide range of strategies and interventions in health promotion. It is important that oral health is considered a priority for both education and health.

Once oral health is recognised as a key area, the next step is to plan the interventions, identifying the strategies that have the most influence on oral and general health, education and development. In order to maximise the impact, it is necessary to integrate the oral health interventions with other health promotion activities.

Interventions should empower students, parents, teachers and community members to make healthy decisions, practise healthy behaviours and create conditions and school environments conductive to health. Health-Promoting Schools involve members of the school and community in planning programmes that respond to their needs and that can be maintained and sustained with available resources and commitments.

It is essential to work with the Parent/Teacher Association (PTA), where appropriate. However, experiences worldwide have shown that two important groups may be very helpful in creating a Health-Promoting School, namely a School Health Team and Community Advisory Committee. A School Health Team is a designated group of people who are committed to work together to promote the health of all people who are working and learning at school.

Depending on local circumstances, it should comprise a balance of representatives, including students, parents, school governors, teachers and school staff, members of teachers' representative organisations, PTA representatives, administrators, food service providers and health care providers. Ideally, the School Health Team should have between 8 and 14 members.

While it may not be possible to recruit all representatives in some schools, it is recommended that the Team should always include the school principal, at least one teacher and one parent, a health care provider and students. The Team is responsible for the management, co-ordination and monitoring of health promotion policies and action plans and for establishing links with district education personnel, local health officials and provincial or national network or ministry-level staff. It also provides leadership, communication and support to school staff and community members and arranges training where necessary.

If a school does not have a School Health Team, oral health promotion can provide a useful impetus for its formation, a model on which other health promoting activities may be based. Given that schools should implement programmes that are responsive to local needs, it is important that students, parents, school governors and school staff including teachers and management are consulted from the outset. Active participation provides a sense of ownership, a vital element of successful programmes.

Teachers and other school staff can help ensure that programmes are developed with consideration to their existing knowledge, skills and abilities, as well as training needs. Given the availability of resources and local circumstances, their input is crucial for ensuring that strategies and interventions are practical, realistic and achievable.

The School Health Team should be given time, resources, authority and support to lead and oversee health promotion activities in school. Each member or a sub-group of members, while working with the whole of the School Health Team, can have designated special responsibility for a given task. For example, an Oral Health Sub-Committee may be formed to address oral health and related issues.

The Community Advisory Committee consists of members or leaders in the wider community who are best able to advise and provide support to the school. They understand the key oral health related issues affecting the community and school, have access to resources that can contribute to health promotion and have a significant influence on creating a supportive environment for oral health.

Committee members foster good relationships between the school and the community at large, strengthening the impact of oral health promotion interventions. Working closely with the School Health Team, the Community Advisory Committee can help:

— advocate the development of a Health-Promoting School with leaders, staff and members of their own organisations and agencies;

— outreach to all parts of the community, lobbying for support;

— encourage other community groups to become

involved in oral health issues and interventions, strengthening community participation;

— *identify and obtain resources for projects and activities;*

— *help assess oral health problems and opportunities that affect the community.*

The Community Advisory Committee should include men and women with a wide range of expertise and skills who are:

— *interested in, and committed to, oral health and health promotion in general;*

— *knowledgeable about the community;*

— *influential in the community or district;*

— *capable of mobilising support and connections;*

— *representative of the local community in terms of geographical, social, economic, cultural and religious composition.*

Potential partners include families, youth, health service providers and representatives of trade unions, women's groups, early childhood education, local government, arts and crafts societies, banking, sanitation/public works, law enforcement, local businesses, transportation, NGOs, charities and development organisations. In some communities, it may not be possible to form two separate groups for the School Health Team and Community Advisory Committee.

To support the development of an effective oral health promotion effort, policy- and decision-makers and other interested groups should consider conducting a situation analysis, a process that involves the collection and analysis of relevant information from a variety of sources. The aim of the situation analysis is to assess the needs, resources and conditions that are relevant to the planning and development of a Health-Promoting School.

Schools can help foster healthy public policies. Policies that are useful in promoting oral health include:

- *oral health education within the school curriculum;*
- *oral hygiene;*
- *sugar and healthy eating policies including canteen, tuck shops, vending machines;*
- *violence and bullying;*
- *trauma and emergency care;*
- *fluorides (e.g. milk or water fluoridation, affordable toothpaste and mouthrinse);*
- *safe water and sanitation;*
- *infection control;*
- *safe environment;*
- *HIV/AIDS;*
- *Exercise;*
- *smoking and tobacco use;*
- *alcohol;*
- *substance abuse.*

The development and maintenance of oral health interventions as part of a Health-Promoting School are influenced by the level of support from the local community. It is crucial that parents and community members are consulted in the design, planning, delivery, content and evaluation of school oral health promotion initiatives from the outset.

Community participation is particularly important to ensure the issues are addressed adequately and effectively, creating a sense of community ownership. More importantly, such involvement maximises the potential of expertise, facilities and resources that are available. Community group meetings, PTAs, formal presentations, open houses, civic clubs and religious centres are useful for promoting and encouraging community participation.

Supportive school policies are essential components of a Health-Promoting School. Policies should be brief and simple documents that provide a supportive framework, detailing the rationale, objectives and guidelines for the development, implementation and evaluation of oral health promotion activities in schools, made available. If preferred, a single policy document that covers all elements, areas and activities of a Health-Promoting School can be developed.

Alternatively, a number of specific or individual policies can be generated, for example in relation to the school environment, behaviour/lifestyle and curriculum. Nonetheless, they should take into account local factors and resources and, more importantly, incorporate input from students, parents, teachers, administrators and all relevant members of the school community. They should also consider the key oral health issues and concerns, reflecting the needs, priorities and cultural preferences of the school and local community.

Collaboration and coordination between health, education and food and agricultural departments of the *government and between the school and the community are crucial in planning policy. Coherent policies and legislation across sectors are needed to avoid contradictory and unacceptable policies. They should be reviewed and evaluated regularly, ensuring that all components of a Health-Promoting School are addressed.*

Policies regarding a Health-Promoting School environment, health education and training for teachers are particularly important for oral health promotion. For example, school policies should make healthy eating the easier choice and ensure that sanitation and safe water are adequately provided in school.

The following guidelines could be included in the formulation of an oral health policy:

— *Teachers, parents, students and all other relevant school personnel are involved in the planning, development and review process;*

— *The School Health Team and Community Advisory Committee meet periodically to review development and maintain coordination between the school and community;*

— *The school curriculum includes oral health in the school health education programme and as an integral part of other relevant subject areas, such as personal development, maths, biology, chemistry and social science;*

— *Teachers and other school staff receive systematic and ongoing training in oral health and prevention of oral diseases;*

— *The school canteen, cafeterias, snack bars, tuck shops*

and vending machines serve nutritious foods and drinks that are conducive to good oral health. School canteen staff and food providers are educated about diet and oral health;

— *If feasible and appropriate, the school considers school-based public health preventive interventions such as water and milk fluoridation;*

— *The school ensures that sufficient facilities are available for oral health activities in school and the premises are adequately safe to prevent craniofacial trauma;*

— *The school ensures that there is appropriate accident prevention policy and practice in school;*

— *In case of emergency, clear protocol is provided to ensure vital actions are taken without delay;*

— *The school monitors oral health related injuries, sickness and absenteeism;*

— *Working with the school health services, the school assesses the oral health status of students regularly and ensures that students have access to oral health care services. Teachers are trained to undertake certain screening and assessment procedures;*

— *The school plays a key role in advocating and lobbying for water fluoridation in areas of poor dental health and for the availability of affordable fluoride toothpaste;*

— *School health services offer screening and treatment for oral disease and work collaboratively with the school staff, parents and the community to promote oral health;*

— *Parents are educated about the value of good oral health and essential oral health practices at home.*

They are encouraged to take an active role in school committees and participate in oral health activities and programmes in school and the community. Teachers and school staff play a fundamental role in carrying out day-to-day oral health promotion activities and interventions. It is important to engage them early in the design and planning stages. A staff meeting is a useful forum for stimulating their interest.

Role of Parents

Parents influence their children's oral health directly by providing a home environment that is conducive to oral health. Through primary socialisation, they convey norms and serve as role models. Their input in monitoring children's oral hygiene practices and dietary behaviours at home is paramount. Given that parents play a key role in promoting sustainable healthy oral health behaviours at home, their involvement and commitment are essential.

Parents and other significant family members should be educated about the importance of oral health, consequences of oral diseases and preventive oral health practices. They should be encouraged to take an active role in their children's oral health, reinforcing and complementing school efforts to promote good oral health behaviours and conditions that reduce the risk of oral diseases. Parental support can be mobilised through PTA, school governors and, if necessary, special meetings at school.

The goals provide a focus for action and should describe, in broad terms, what the programme will achieve. The goals of oral health promotion in a Health-Promoting School should include, but not be limited to, the following aims:

— *To provide a physical, organisational and psychosocial school environment that is conducive to oral health of students, teachers and school staff, as well as families and the community;*

— *To reduce the risk factors associated with oral health;*

— *To improve oral health knowledge and attitudes;*

— *To develop skills and behaviours for good oral health.*

The goals are then broken into specific outcome and process objectives so that it is clear what needs to be done, when and why. Objectives are explicit targets to be met in order to achieve the goals. They should be specific, measurable, achievable and appropriate but challenging, realistic and be set within a specified and reasonable time frame. It may be useful to divide the objectives into short-term, intermediate and long-term objectives, depending on local circumstances and the nature of the problems.

A Health Promoting School strives to use the school's full organisational capacity to improve the health of students, school staff, families and community members. Such a school offers many opportunities to promote oral health as an integral part of health and well being.

Oral health promotion interventions can be used as an entry point for the development and enhancement of policies, planning groups and various components that serve as a framework for Health-Promoting Schools. Comprehensive school programmes should include:

- *Healthy school environment;*
- *School health education;*
- *School health services;*
- *Nutrition and food services;*
- *Physical education and sport;*
- *Mental health and well being;*
- *Health promotion for school staff;*
- *School and community relationships and collaboration.*

The effectiveness of interventions integrated into each of the components is determined by how they are supported by people, policies and trained staff. The effectiveness is also influenced by the extent to which interventions in each of these components integrate and complement with other health promotion efforts.

Not all schools will have the resources to incorporate oral health into all components at the same time. Each school has to establish its own priorities. A Health-Promoting School enables all parties concerned - students, parents, teachers and school staff, and community members -to work together to set the priorities and to decide how and the extent to which the components should be addressed. It may be more important, if not more feasible technically and financially, to start with small changes than to address all components simultaneously.

Each school needs to assess what is realistically achievable, progressively building on strategies that work to maximise the full potential of a Health-Promoting School. School environment determines the effectiveness and sustainability of oral health promotion interventions. Supportive school environment enables students and school staff to develop their physical, mental and social potential, enhancing the relationships between members of the school community.

Supportive environment encourages healthy lifestyles and behaviours that are conducive to oral health, making healthier choice the easier choice. In a Health-Promoting School, much emphasis is placed on the supportive school environment, both physical and psychosocial. The physical and psychosocial school environments should be coherent with, and supportive of, each other.

The physical environment includes the location and surroundings of the school, school grounds, buildings, classrooms, eating facilities and other structural features. The condition of the physical environment and policies regarding its use can have a significant impact on oral health directly as well as indirectly through lifestyles and oral health behaviours. The school should be located in a safe environment, away from busy roads, dangerous industrial sites and polluted areas.

The cleanliness of the premises, sufficient provision of rubbish disposal, safe water, hygienic sanitary facilities and structurally safe and well designed school buildings and playgrounds are only the basics, but without which other developments cannot be progressed. The physical environment of the local community in which the school is situated may also form part of the school environment.

The following examples of oral health-related

aspects of a healthy physical environment, supported by appropriate healthy policies, can be considered.

— *Safe water and sanitation: The provision of clean and safe water, sufficient sanitary facilities and adequate waste collection and disposal is essential to good health and well being. These facilities are also fundamental to good oral health. They are essential to oral health promotion activities such as toothbrushing drills at lunchtime. Good sanitation and waste disposal facilities reduce the risk of infection. In some developing countries, many households may not have safe and clean water supply and sanitation; the school may be the only place where children can clean their teeth. If the school has not already been equipped with these basic facilities, oral health promotion can be used as an impetus for the school to install them.*

— *Healthy dietary practices: A healthy environment supports the adoption of healthy lifestyles. With the canteens, tuck shops and vending machines providing healthy foods and drinks, supported by healthy policies, the practice of healthy oral health behaviours is more sustainable. Promoting good dietary behaviours also reinforces other health messages in school, such as healthy nutrition, healthy heart and cancer prevention.*

— *Health supportive environment: A pleasant school environment with spacious and comfortable surroundings enhances physical, mental and social health and promotes healthy behaviours. Apart from policies governing vending machines, tuck shops and canteens, a no smoking or smokeless tobacco policy is critical to good oral health, most notably for periodontal health and oral cancer prevention. Creating a tobacco-free school requires the full support and commitment from everyone concerned. Safe school interior structures, buildings and playgrounds reduce the risk of dental trauma. With appropriate dental first aid and trauma policies, vital actions can be taken to avoid permanent tooth loss, if accidents occur.*

— *Outside vendors: Surroundings outside the school premises also need to be conducive to health, in order to avoid sending conflicting messages to students. It may be necessary to educate, if not impose restrictions on, food vendors and kiosk traders in or near the school premises to offer nutritious foods and drinks that are conducive to oral health. The sale of sweets, soft drinks and tobacco containing products to students in the vicinity of school should be prohibited.*

The psychosocial environment refers to the social and psychological conditions that underpin health and education potential of the school community. The school culture and organisational structure influence the psychosocial environment. Stress can inflate interpersonal conflicts and violent behaviours and can lead to smoking, excessive alcohol consumption and the use of comfort foods that are high in sugar, factors that increase the risk of oral disease.

This is particularly relevant in today's societies with prevailing social and family problems where stress can affect all ages. A supportive social culture helps ameliorate the stress experienced by students and staff; which in turn improves their oral health.

Children's social, personal and life experiences and interaction at home, in school and the society have a significant impact on their oral health and health development in general. The primary goals of school oral health education are to help children develop personal lifelong skills, raise health consciousness, improve understanding and healthy attitudes, to promote healthy behaviours, and thereby to reduce risks of oral disease.

School health education can be provided in school as a specific subject or as an integral part of other subjects. It can also be included in extracurricular activities. Ideally, it encompasses a series of planned sequential courses of instruction from primary through secondary school levels, addressing the underlying physical, psychological, cultural and social determinants of oral health, in the context of good general health and well being.

School health education focuses on:

- *important behaviours and conditions that promote oral health or that reduce risk of oral disease;*
- *skills needed to negotiate and practise those behaviours or to address those conditions both personally and collectively;*
- *knowledge, attitudes, beliefs and values related to those behaviours and conditions*
- *learning experiences that allow students to model and practise skills;*
- *personal development;*

— *responsibility at home and in the society.*

In a Health-Promoting School, depending on socio-cultural conditions and resources, oral health promotion should target:

— *maintaining good oral hygiene with daily toothbrushing drills supervised by teachers;*

— *the use of fluoride, including affordable fluoride toothpaste and fluoride rinsing programmes;*

— *promoting good nutrition;*

— *reducing the consumption and frequency of sugary snacks and drinks;*

— *promoting the consumption of fruit and vegetables;*

— *promoting water or milk fluoridation;*

— *promoting regular dental check-ups and care;*

— *preventing or reducing tobacco use, alcohol consumption and substance abuse;*

— *preventing accidents, violence and anti-social behaviours;*

— *taking a wider responsibility at home and in the society.*

In a Health-Promoting School, oral health education should be regularly reinforced at home and further developed in school at key educational stages throughout the children's school career.

A good educational programme utilises a variety of learning and teaching methods, including lectures, seminars, practical experiments, discussions, group work, problem-solving exercises, debates and role-play with appropriate and stimulating visual aids. Self-directed learning encourages students to take responsibility for their learning.

A diversity of instructional strategies is essential to effective curricular development. However, the learning and teaching strategies and materials employed must be appropriate and acceptable to the target students, taking into account the learning objectives and resources available. They should also aim to promote active involvement and reinforcement.

In a Health-Promoting School, oral health education should be an important part of school health education and incorporated across a number of curricular areas, as relevant. Teachers in all disciplines should be encouraged to include oral health in their teaching programmes and activities. They should be inspired to make the curriculum exciting and stimulating for students to acquire good oral health knowledge and behaviours and to make healthy decisions.

When teaching a practical skill such as toothbrushing technique, it is necessary for the teachers to learn, and be competent on brushing their own teeth effectively first. This is particularly important as teachers are often considered as role models by students. Guidelines for teachers in monitoring and supervising toothbrushing drills should be developed.

Given the competing demands in an already fully packed curriculum, some teachers may be too inundated with other curricular activities. In order to promote oral health education in the curriculum, it is imperative for the government and health professionals to provide sustainable support, in terms of technical assistance, funding and/or learning materials. Such a support makes it easier for teachers to consider oral health education in their teaching programmes.

Students play an essential role in the implementation of school oral health programmes. Among many other ways, oral health education can be delivered using peer teaching, a strategy that employs students themselves to act as positive role models and educators for other students. For oral health education, peer leaders can help monitor other students' oral hygiene and develop self-care capacity in oral health.

However, peer leaders must be properly trained to ensure that they have adequate knowledge and skills to support other students and activities. Students may be encouraged to take the initiative to help develop innovative oral health education materials that are used by other students and members of the community.

Participating in community work fosters valuable links with the wider community, helping them fulfil their role in the community. As part of the project work, students can be actively involved in collecting data for evaluation purposes, information that can prove invaluable to the school. School oral health services, part of the school health services, help screen, prevent, control and monitor oral diseases and conditions, as well as maintain good oral health.

They play an important role in oral and general health promotion, supporting the efforts made by the school, teachers and students. In Health-Promoting Schools, the oral health team works collaboratively with the primary health care team to provide accessible oral health services primarily to students. To avoid duplication of efforts, they should be coordinated with other services and activities in school and the community. Models for providing school oral health services vary immensely between, as well as within, developed and developing countries.

While there are comprehensive on-site oral health facilities in schools in some countries (e.g. Denmark), many schools may not be able to provide access to any facilities. Depending on the level of resources available, school oral health services may be provided by the dental team or the school health team and school nurses who have had appropriate dental training. Where resources are stretched, teachers and school staff can be trained to undertake oral health surveillance and first aid duties. However, the role of nurses, health workers, teachers and community workers in relation to the school oral health programme must be carefully monitored and evaluated.

The types and levels of the school oral health services provided are determined by the oral health status of the school population, needs and demand of students, parents, school staff, the community, the local and national health care system and resources (including trained dental staff) available. School oral health services may include screening, diagnosis, needs assessment, clinical preventive oral care and treatment of oral disease, regular monitoring and, for more complicated conditions, and/or referral to other dental or medical specialists and secondary care.

In some developing countries, the provision of emergency care, dental extraction, restorative treatment with atraumatic restorative technique may prove very important. Screening of teeth and mouth enables early detection, and timely interventions towards oral diseases and conditions, leading to substantial cost savings. It plays an important role in the planning and provision of school oral health services as well as health services.

Appropriate and effective efforts can be targeted at those who are at risk or in need. Signs of some general health conditions can be identified through oral health screening, such as malnutrition and diabetes. Oral health screening is not necessarily performed by dentists or dental auxiliaries. It can be effectively carried out by trained school health nurses, school teachers, or community workers.

It can be incorporated into routine general health screening, surveillance programmes or other activities in schools. Oral health screening can form part of the oral and general health education and self care programmes in the school curriculum. Children are receptive to health promotion messages when they are actively involved in the activities that are highly relevant to them, promoting oral health in the context of good general health.

Based on the screening results, students who are in need of care should be referred to the dental team for detailed examination, treatment and follow-up monitoring. Ideally, all school children should, resource permitting, be offered a regular dental check-up. Undoubtedly, in some countries, the school oral health services may not be able to provide all necessary care to all children.

However, the role of the school oral and health services remain significant in the promotion of oral health and general well being. The school oral health services also provide useful facilities for clinical data collection, part of an oral health information system. Such information can prove invaluable to the school in relation to the planning, development and evaluation of the Health-Promoting School.

For the services that cannot be offered in school, the school oral health services can provide referrals to other school services, such as counselling and other general health issues and to local health services, specialist care and other community agencies, as appropriate. Such collaborative working improves communication and promotes partnership between oral health and medical teams, school and the community.

Diet, nutrition and oral health are intricately linked. Micronutrient deficiency, a condition that is common among school-age children in developing countries, and poor dietary practices increase the risk of oral disease. Healthy nutrition interventions with supportive policies are therefore an integral part of a Health-Promoting School that aims to promote oral health.

As part of oral health promotion, schools can enforce healthy snacks or no sugar policies to support healthy eating behaviours, provide nutritious meals and, where necessary, micronutrient supplements. Oral health activities can be included in the assessment and monitoring of nutritional status such as a school height census.

While school food services are often managed by the public or private sectors through the ministry of education, it is important for schools, teachers, students and school oral health services to collaborate closely with them to support healthy eating initiatives in schools.

Physical exercise, sport and leisure activities help maintain physical and mental fitness, a fundamental prerequisite to health and well being. Evidence suggests that physical and mental wellness improves academic performance. Exercise and leisure activities are an important part of stress management. However, there are oral health implications. Sports and physical activities inflate the risk of head and face injuries. Studies have shown that some sport drinks with high acidity that are popular among adolescents can lead to dental erosion. The use of mouth guards should be encouraged in high-risk contact sports to protect teeth.

A Health-Promoting School also promotes the mental health and well being of students and school staff, enabling them to fulfil their physical, social and psychological potential. Poor facial and/or dental appearance may have a negative impact on mental health and well being. Stress, bullying and violence can lead to the consumption of sugary snacks and alcohol, smoking and violent behaviours, which have serious oral health implications.

These issues should be addressed by health promotion, with supportive policies. Students and school staff should be equipped with knowledge and skills that help them prevent and, if unavoidable, deal with interpersonal conflicts; cope with stress, peer pressure and other social forces; and develop self-esteem and confidence. Counselling and support services for students and staff should be available.

A Health-Promoting School places a special emphasis on staff welfare and working conditions, applying the principles and strategies of health promotion to the workplace. Employees and their families along with the organisational, managerial and environmental characteristics of the school are considered. Healthy working conditions and good management and organisational structure can help reduce the stress levels experienced by staff members.

Well-designed and health-orientated classrooms, offices, staff rooms, cooking and dining facilities can be a starting point. Health promoting facilities including those designed for exercise and relaxation are imperative. Staff morale and workload must be carefully monitored to avoid the risk of burnout.

Oral health education materials together with other health messages should be prominent throughout the school including staff rooms. A tobacco-free school, if feasible and supported by staff, is one of the most effective strategies for providing smoke-free working environment. However, support services that help the staff members deal with stress, give up smoking or tobacco use or lose weight should be available.

As part of in-service training, a tailored-made oral health promotion programme that aims at providing knowledge and influencing attitudes and behaviours should be available regularly, helping staff members acquire and sustain healthy lifestyles. Teachers and school staff are encouraged to identify essential policies and practices and to work with the School Health Team, parents and the local community collaboratively to promote oral health and general well being in school and the community.

The community is a critical component of a Health-

Promoting School. Community members should feel that the school is approachable and receptive to their contribution and, more importantly, that they are valued. A Health-Promoting School provides a valuable link between the school, parents and the community, promoting joint working to support the development and implementation of oral health promotion initiatives. Family and community members can be involved in the following ways:

— *Taking part in the planning and decision making process, such as taking part in the School Health Team and Community Advisory Committee;*

— *Participating in school-led oral health activities at school and in the community, such as Oral Health Day, exhibitions and health fairs;*

— *Providing support and resources, in terms of skills, expertise, materials and funding;*

— *Advocating oral health including lobbying for healthy environment and water fluoridation.*

A Health Promoting School collaborates with parents and families to ensure oral health promotion efforts are reinforced at home. Parents are important role models that help shape children's development and influence their lifestyles. Parents are responsible for providing pack lunches and, in many developing countries, toothbrushes for their children to use in schools. It is important that these foods, drinks and oral hygiene aids are conducive to oral and general health.

Schools can serve as a focal point, providing essential training and health education materials for parents and families. Parents are educated about their own oral health as well as caring for other members of the family. Educational programmes are most effective when parents and families meet together and support each other at regular meetings in schools.

Good communication between school oral health services and parents is of paramount importance. Equally, students are encouraged to impart the knowledge and skills that are beneficial to other family members. For those who do not attend schools, outreach programmes that involve using parents and family members as facilitators can help promote oral health to these families and entice them to be part of the school community.

Community collaboration can strengthen interventions to promote better oral health. Successful partnership builds on trust, respect, effective communication, shared mission and resource coordination. The school and community partners can benefit from each other. There may be a wide range of organisations and local businesses with which collaboration can be fostered. For example, food traders, manufacturers and businesses, water companies, commercial organisations and toothpaste manufacturers and retailers should be encouraged to:

- *promote healthy eating, foods and drinks that are low in sugar, salt and fat;*
- *offer financial support for oral health promotion programmes and campaigns; advice on healthy lifestyle, relevant visits to their stores and, where appropriate, oral health advice;*
- *supply water with optimal level of fluoride;*

— *provide healthy choices;*

— *provide clear and accurate labelling of foods, drinks and healthcare products;*

— *provide and promote the sale of affordable toothpaste with fluoride as well as good quality toothbrushes;*

— *provide educational materials for school oral health programmes.*

The mass media can be used effectively to promote oral health. Information can be distributed efficiently through mass media. For example, a television programme that involves using popular icons or idols can be employed to promote oral health messages. Undoubtedly, such a high profile campaign can raise awareness. However, these campaigns can be costly and supplementary activities are needed to promote awareness, knowledge gain and behaviour change.

Nonetheless, the media may be educated and encouraged to stop targeting children and adolescents in advertising products that may increase the risk of oral disease, e.g. smoking and smokeless tobacco, sugary foods and drinks.

Growth of Child Nutrition

Working with parents and families to improve nutrition is one of the most important ways in which health workers can promote child health, especially in those developing countries where resources are very limited. Understanding the cycle of malnutrition and the need for a life cycle approach is the first step to improving nutrition. A child who is undernourished does not grow well and is more prone to infection.

Frequent infections affect nutrient absorption and cause loss of appetite, which in turn means a child eats less. This is the start of the malnutrition/infection cycle. Andrew Tomkins looks at nutrition interventions that can help improve immunity and reduce the risk of infection.

Severely malnourished children need special care and attention. Where referral to hospital is not possible, appropriate treatment at health centre level can help save lives. Breastfeeding is one of the most important aspects of childhood nutrition but in many countries exclusive breastfeeding is rare. Isatou Semega-Janneh describes how a project in The Gambia provided community support to mothers to help them exclusively breastfeed.

Iron deficiency anaemia is the most common nutritional deficiency in the world. In many populations the amount of iron absorbed from the diet is not enough to meet requirements, especially during infancy and pregnancy. Health workers often find it difficult to spend time counselling individual parents and families about good nutrition. For this reason it is important to involve women's groups and other community members in activities that improve child nutrition.

Current advice is to avoid any other fluids other than breastmilk for newborn babies to encourage exclusive breastfeeding. But some mothers do not produce enough breastmilk early enough which can lead to newborn hypoglycaemia. A day old child brought to my clinic with signs of hypoglycaemia would have died, had we not quickly given him 50 per cent dextrose solution. The risk of hypoglycaemia can be reduced, by starting exclusive breastfeeding within 30-60 minutes of delivery.

The early milk (colostrum) especially important. Where customs lead to a delayed start or infrequent breastfeeds, hypoglycaemia requiring immediate intervention may follow. Use of dextrose solution is justified, but intravenous administration of a 10% solution is more effective than oral treatment. The newborn should discharged only after careful examination for any abnormality and when exclusive and effective breastfeeding has been established.

The term Protein Energy Malnutrition (PEM) misleading. Protein is only one of several nutrients that may be low in the diets of children who grow poorly. For example, many of these children may be deficient in nutrients such as potassium or zinc, as well as energy. The use of the term PEM results in some health workers, understandably, promoting 'high protein foods' such eggs, instead of a 'good mixed' diet.

In rural areas, clinic's main problem with referral is lack of money. Carers have to convince heads of household that referral and funds are needed and then find the cash. Sometimes after our emergency treatment a sick child seems 'better' and parents do not see the need for more diagnostic tests or treatment to prevent complications. Or they may take the child to hospital several days later when her condition has changed.

Each year more than one out of every ten babies in developing countries are born full term but have low birth weight (LBW). LBW babies are at risk of:

— illness and death from infections, especially pneumonia and diarrhoea

— growing poorly

— impaired mental development

— developing chronic disease when adults.

Maternal undernutrition is the main reason for poor foetal growth. A woman is underweight if she weighs less than 45kg or has an upper mid-arm circumference of less than 23cm. If a woman is likely to become pregnant soon give her iron/folic acid tablets and, if possible, iodine supplements if iodised salt is not available.

Pregnant women encourage them to eat an additional small meal each day. For example, porridge with milk, bananas and groundnuts, or a chapati and dhal. Give iron/folic acid tablets. Start at first contact visit during pregnancy. Give low dose vitamin A if they are at high risk of vitamin A deficiency. High doses (50,000 IU/week or over) may harm the foetus. Discuss with women and their families how women can reduce workloads in late pregnancy. Women who have just given birth.

Encourage exclusive breastfeeding for about six months. Later advise about complementary feeding and then how to feed children when breastfeeding stops. Advise them to eat an additional 'good mixed meal' each day while breastfeeding. Give one high dose of vitamin A within eight weeks of delivery (or within six weeks if not breastfeeding).

Continue giving iron and folic acid if a woman is anaemic. Give women and their partners information on

HIV prevention and child spacing. Explain to parents of older children that:

- *School-age children need about three meals and two snacks each day containing a variety of foods, especially foods supplying iron.*
- *Adolescents need extra food and nutrients, especially iron as they are growing fast.*
- *'Slimming' should be discouraged as this might cause undernutrition.*
- *Adolescent girls who become pregnant risk becoming under-nourished as they are still growing.*

Malnutrition is a significant underlying factor in more than half the deaths of young children in developing countries. This is particularly true for deaths from diarrhoea, measles, acute respiratory infection, meningitis and malaria. Malnutrition impairs the immune system so that infections are more frequent, more serious and last longer. Programmes for the prevention and early treatment of childhood illness include several key nutritional interventions. Such as:

- *reducing the prevalence of low birth weight, for example by using the lifecyle approach to nutrition*
- *improving infant feeding and complementary feeding*
- *preventing micronutrient deficiences.*

Breastfeeding, particularly exclusive breastfeeding, reduces the number of infections and deaths in infants. In developing countries, non-breastfed infants are three to four times more likely to die in the first three months of life. The risks are particularly high where environmental contamination and risk of diarrhoea and respiratory infection is common.

Breastfeeding also protects older infants, for example, breastfed infants aged between four to eight months are 60-90 percent less likely to die from infectious diseases. Breastmilk contains live cells and immunoglobins which give babies immunity to many infections.

Tragically, breastmilk can transmit HIV. In some situations, where hygiene is good, mothers are well informed and the family can afford an appropriate breastmilk substitute, the risk of infant death from an HIV-related infection acquired through breastmilk is much greater than the risk of infection from not being breast-fed.

However, in many situations, the use of breastmilk substitutes is extremely hazardous and carries a higher risk than breastfeeding. Recent studies suggest that for the first three months, HIV-positive mothers who breastfeed exclusively are less likely to transmit HIV to their infants compared with those who either 'mixed feed' or never breastfeed.

A number of women in poor countries develop subclinical mastitis. This tends to increase the number of inflammatory cells and HIV viruses in breastmilk. Therefore prevention of mastitis may be an important way of reducing transmission of HIV through breastmilk.

Children who grow poorly are more likely to suffer from serious infections or to die. Detect growth faltering early by regularly monitoring growth, especially in the first year. Prevent poor growth and improve immunity *by giving good food to children over six months to complement and, later, replace breastmilk.*

Many micronutrients are needed for a healthy immune system. Vitamin A deficiency depresses the immune system. In areas where vitamin A deficiency is common, young children are thirty per cent more likely to die. Giving a high dose of vitamin A to children between six months and five years reduces deaths. Special attention should be given to children with measles and xerophthalmia.

Vitamin A supplementation does not improve the clinical outcome of children with pneumonia or acute watery diarrhoea. Its effect on dysentery and persistent diarrhoea needs further research. A recent study in Papua New Guinea showed a beneficial effect of vitamin A on malaria. Another study in Nepal found that giving low doses of vitamin A to women who were pregnant, or about to become pregnant, reduced maternal deaths by half.

However, vitamin A does not appear to prevent mother-to-child transmission of HIV. Improving the amount of vitamin A in the diet is the best long-term way to reduce vitamin A deficiency. The best sources are animal foods such as liver, red palm oil and orange fruits and vegetables. The bioavailability of vitamin A from green leaves is less than originally thought. Oils and fats increase absorption.

Children who are zinc-deficient have more episodes of infection, particularly diarrhoea and respiratory disease. Zinc deficiency causes increased losses of intestinal fluid during diarrhoea and delayed recovery from acute or persistent diarrhoea. If a two week course of a cheap syrup containing zinc acetate (2mgs of elemental zinc per kg/day) is given to these children:

— *recovery from diarrhoea is faster*

— *purging is less*

— *there are fewer episodes of*

— *diarrhoea in the following months.*

Zinc deficiency is common because the best sources of zinc are fish and meat, which are often too expensive for many families. The bioavailability in plant foods, such as cereals, is low. At present, the recommendation is to give zinc supplements during treatment of severely malnourished children particularly those with persistent diarrhoea and acute diarrhoea.

Zinc deficiency is an important cause of low birth weight in malnourished populations. Supplementation of zinc-deficient women during pregnancy improves weight gain and birth weight but accurate detection of zinc deficiency is difficult.

Iron circulates freely in the blood in healthy children and is eaten by bacteria during septicaemia. For this reason iron supplements should not be given to children with an infection or severe malnutrition, because of the risk of increasing the severity of infection. However, since iron deficiency can depress immunity it is important to prevent anaemia in women and children and so avoid the need for large, potentially dangerous, doses of iron supplements.

There has been concern that iron supplements might increase malaria episodes or severity. However, a recent analysis of all studies showed that giving oral iron supplements to people in malarious areas does not necessarily increase malaria parasitaemia and does not increase clinical episodes. Therefore it is recommended that oral iron supplements are given in areas where malaria is endemic and iron deficiency anaemia prevalent.

There have been many accounts of people with rickets (due to vitamin D deficiency) being more susceptible to tuberculosis. Improving vitamin D status may be one way of helping to prevent tuberculosis, and possibly other infections such as pneumonia.

Vitamin D status is improved by exposing children to sunlight and giving vitamin D-rich foods (such as egg yolk, fortified margarine). Referral to hospital should be the first choice for severely malnourished children but is sometimes impossible.

Admit if there is visible severe wasting (marasmus) and/or oedema. Look for accompanying conditions such as dehydration or infections. Frequent feeding prevents death from hypoglycaemia and hypothermia and starts to repair the child's body. Feed the child every three hours day and night. Explain to the carer that the child must be fed small amounts slow-ly and persistently. Feed lost through vomiting or dribbling must be replaced.

Keep the child warm and dry to prevent death from hypothermia. Clothe the child (including a hat) and cover with a blanket. Let the child sleep cuddled up to the carer.

Start antibiotics immediately because infections are common and the usual signs are often absent. If the child has no specific signs of infection, give oral cotrimoxazole (5ml paediatric suspension twice daily) for five days.

If the child looks sickly, give ampicillin IM/IV (50mg/kg every six hours) for two days and then amoxycillin orally (15mg/kg every eight hours) for five days and gentamicin IM/IV (7.5mg/kg once a day) for seven days.

If the child does not improve within two days or if gentamicin is not available, add oral chloramphenicol (25mg/kg every eight hours) for five days. If these antibiotics are not available give IM antibiotics such as procaine penicillin and combine them with oral cotrimoxazole.

In high risk areas, treat for malaria using local guidelines. Give a high dose of vitamin A on day one (50,000 IU if aged less than six months, 100,000 IU if aged 6-12 months, 200,000 IU if aged more than 12 months). If there are signs of xerophthalmia, give another high dose on day two and another after two weeks.

Give multivitamins daily if available. Do not give iron until the child's appetite returns as iron makes infections worse. Give extra potassium, magnesium, zinc and copper. If unavailable, give half a tablet/kg of crushed Slow K (potassium) daily. Or prepare potassium solution by putting a teaspoon of fresh cool wood ash in a clean cloth and pouring a cup of cooled boiled water through it.

Potassium is essential for recovery. If you suspect the child is HIV-positive treat associated conditions and try to arrange counselling for his or her parents. Many HIV-positive children can recover from malnutrition although it may take longer than usual. Immunise the child against measles if there is no record that it has been given.

Dehydration is difficult to diagnose in severely malnourished children as malnutrition can also cause the usual signs of sunken eyes, lethargy, and 'slow' skin pinch. Suspect dehydrat-ion if a child has diarrhoea, is thirsty or not passing urine. Do not use IV rehydration unless a child is shocked as too much fluid can cause heart failure. Because the child has excess sodium, give diluted oral rehydration solution:

Mix the ORS sachet with two litres water and add 50g sugar. Add potassium and magnesium if available. If there are no ORS sachets, use eight rounded teaspoons of sugar and half a teaspoon of salt in one litre of clean water. Also add 20ml of the electrolyte solution, if available. Rehydrate slowly and monitor the child carefully. If the child's breathing and heart rate increase, too much fluid has been given. If this happens, stop and reassess after one hour.

Signs of recovery are loss of oedema, increased appetite and improved mood. This usually occurs after two to seven days. Then:

— *Change to an energy/nutrient-rich diet but continue giving potassium. Give other electrolytes and micronutrients if available.*

— *Give iron (3mg/kg/day).*

— *Teach the carer how to stimulate the child, to encourage mental as well as physical catch-up.*

It may now be safe to discharge the child if she or he can be closely monitored. Before discharge:

— *Discuss with the family how to give a good mixed*

diet and care for the child at home.

— Ask the carer to bring the child back at least weekly for check-ups, possible.

— Check the child is fully immunised.

— Try to deal with the underlying reasons for the child becoming malnourished.

There is growing concern about the increase in child obesity as well as adult obesity in developing countries. A recent study in Thailand found a 12-16 per cent increase in obesity in school-age children over two years. Obese children often become obese adults. Obesity, especially abdominal obesity increases the risk of conditions such as coronary heart disease, non-insulin dependant diabetes mellitus and hypertension in adulthood.

There is now strong evidence that undernutrition in the womb and in early childhood increases the risk of obesity and related disorders in later life. For example, during the 2 nd World War there was an imposed famine in the Netherlands. Children born to mothers who were in the first six months of pregnancy during the famine, had a higher incidence of obesity at the age of 18 years. Some studies have found that:

— Low weight and size at birth (due to maternal malnutrition) increased the risk of a range of chronic non-communicable diseases such as coronary heart disease, hypertension and non-insulin dependant diabetes in later life.

— In developing countries there seems to be a close link between an increase in stunting in the population and the growing epidemic of obesity. Slower growth in height may lead to the laying down of more body fat.

— As children recover from malnutrition there are alterations in body composition. The ratio of fat to

4

School Feeding: Towards Effective Education

Today, the environment in which School Feeding Programs (SFPs) operate is quite different than even a decade ago, and significantly different from several decades ago, when many of the on-going SFPs were initiated. World food resources are dwindling, increasing the competition for food aid, while the use of public sector resources for feeding programs is being more carefully scrutinized. Against this backdrop of potentially more limited resources, the gains in child survival have made it clear that the school-age group requires attention.

SFPs have gained a reputation over the years for being expensive, fraught with implementation problems and ineffective in meeting health, nutrition or educational objectives. This reputation may not be completely unfounded, and in reality the impact of SFPs is uncertain at best, since little work has been done on evaluating them. Until recently, SFPs were viewed as predominantly nutrition/feeding interventions aimed at improving the nutrition status of schoolchildren, so the effects of SFPs on educational outcomes were often not emphasized or examined.

An exception is the recognition of the role that SFPs play in encouraging school enrolment and attendance, an objective that continues to be important in some countries today. Nutritional and health status are powerful influences on a child's learning and on how well a child performs in school. Children who lack certain nutrients in their diet (particularly iron and iodine), or who suffer from protein-energy malnutrition, hunger, parasitic infections or other diseases, do not have the same potential for learning as healthy and well-nourished children.

Weak health and poor nutrition among school-age children diminish their cognitive development either through physiological changes or by reducing their ability to participate in learning experiences - or both. Contrary to conventional wisdom, nutritional status does not improve with age. The extra demands on school-age children (to perform chores, for example, or walk long distances to school) create a need for energy that is much greater than that of younger children.

Moreover, deficiencies of critical nutrients such as iodine, vitamin A and iron among the school-aged are pervasive. It is estimated that 60 million school-age children suffer from iodine deficiency disorders and that another 85 million are at risk for acute respiratory disease and other infections because they are deficient in vitamin A. The number suffering from iron deficiency anemia is greater still - 210 million.

Parasitic worms that infect the intestines or the

blood are a major source of disease and malnutrition in school-age children. An estimated 320 million school-age children are infected with roundworm, 233 million with whipworm, and 239 million with hookworm. Schistosomiasis affects an estimated 200 million people throughout the world, approximately 88 million of whom are under 15 years old. Poor nutrition and health among schoolchildren contributes to the inefficiency of the educational system.

Children with diminished cognitive abilities and sensory impairments naturally perform less well and are more likely to repeat grades and to drop out of school than children who are not impaired; they also enroll in school at a later age, if at all, and finish fewer years of schooling. The irregular school attendance of malnourished and unhealthy children is one of the key factors in poor performance.

Even temporary hunger, common in children who are not fed before going to school, can have an adverse effect on learning. Children who are hungry have more difficulty concentrating and performing complex tasks, even if otherwise well nourished. Improving nutrition and health can lead to better performance, fewer repeated grades and reduced drop out. SFPs are one of several interventions that can address some of the nutrition and health problems of school-age children. SFPs, and other school-based nutrition and health programs, can also motivate parents to enroll their children in school and to see that they attend regularly. Properly designed and effectively implemented SFPs can:

— *Alleviate short-term hunger in malnourished or otherwise well-nourished schoolchildren. This helps to increase the attention and concentration of students producing gains in cognitive function and learning.*

- *Motivate parents to enroll their children in school and have them attend regularly. When programs effectively reduce absenteeism and increase the duration of schooling, educational outcomes (performance, dropout, and repetition) improve.*
- *Address specific micronutrient deficiencies in school-age children. Most important of these are iodine and iron, which directly affect cognition. Meeting the iron and iodine needs of school-age children can translate into better school performance.*
- *Increase community involvement in schools, particularly where programs depend on the community to prepare and serve meals to children. Schools with their communities behind them are more effective than schools with less community involvement.*

The number of hungry school-age children is unknown, but is likely to be a significant problem in various circumstances. Many factors contribute to hunger in schoolchildren : the long distances children have to travel to school, cultural meal practices that include no or small breakfasts or a lack of family time or resources to provide adequate meals to children before and/or during the school day.

Simply alleviating this hunger in schoolchildren helps them to perform better in school. In Jamaica providing breakfast to primary school students significantly increased attendance and arithmetic scores. The children who benefited most were those who were wasted, stunted, or previously malnourished. A US study showed the benefits of providing breakfast to disadvantaged primary school students. Before the start of a school breakfast program, eligible (low-income) children scored significantly lower on achievement testes than those not eligible.

Once in the program, however, the test scores of the children participating in the program improved more than the scores of non-participants. The attendance of participating children also improved. In Peru 23 malnourished and 29 well-nourished 9 to 11 year old boys were studied to assess the effects of breakfast on cognitive performance. Each boy served as his own control in a manner comparable to the Jamaica study cited above.

Breakfast was a nutritionally fortified beverage and a baked grain product fortified with iron, similar to the meal provided in the government-sponsored school breakfast program. A series of cognitive tests were administered in an experimental setting. Speed in performing a short-term memory test and discrimination of geometric patterns were improved under the breakfast condition in both groups. The effect was more pronounced in the nutritionally disadvantaged children.

Children in poor health start school later in life or not at all. A study in Nepal found that the probability of attending school was 5% for stunted children versus 27% for children of normal nutritional status. In Ghana malnourished children entered school at a later age and completed fewer years of school than better nourished children. The number of days that a child attends school is related to cognition and performance.

SFPs can have a positive effect on rates of enrollment and attendance. A recent evaluation of an on-going school feeding program in Burkina Faso found that school canteens were associated with increased school enrollment, regular attendance, consistently lower repeater rates, lower dropout rates in disadvantaged provinces, and higher success rates on national exams, especially among girls.

A small pilot school feeding program in Malawi was evaluated for its effect on enrollment and attendance. Over a three month period there was a 5% increase in enrollment and up to 36% improvement in attendance/absenteeism compared to control schools over the same period. Niger has one of the five lowest school enrollment rates in the world; the school feeding program is intended to enhance attendance of nomad and transhumant families, particularly of girls.

Beneficiaries receive the equivalent of the total daily recommended food intake in three meals per day. In addition, as an incentive for girls' participation in schools, some families receive an additional take-home ration. Evidence from past experience with the SFP shows that it contributes to its objectives: whenever canteens have been closed, even provisionally, immediate and high absenteeism follows and children are withdrawn from school. In areas with nomadic and transhumant populations, the school year cannot commence until food stocks arrive.

Although not a school feeding program in the traditional sense, school-based food distribution has also been used successfully to improve enrollment and attendance among school-age children, particularly girls. In Bangladesh a program of school-based food distribution increased enrollment by 20% versus a 2% decline in non-participating schools. In Pakistan, a program provides an income transfer in the form of one or two tins of oil to families whose girls attend school for 20 days per month.

These food transfer mechanisms do not offer the same potential benefits, for example, meeting short-term hunger and specific nutritional needs, as programs that deliver food directly to beneficiaries. These kinds of programs should therefore be assessed within the context of other food and resource transfer programs.

Deficiencies of iron and iodine are among the most harmful types of malnutrition with regard to cognition. Iron deficiency renders children listless, inattentive and uninterested in learning. The research literature suggests a causal link between iron deficiency anemia and less than optimal behavior for learning.

Poor performance on a wide range of achievement tests among iron deficient children in school has been consistently documented. Remediation of iron deficiency through supplementation has eliminated the differences in school performance and IQ scores between schoolchildren previously deficient in iron and those without iron deficiencies.

In the case of iodine, most studies have focussed on the differences in cognitive test performance between children who lived in communities with and without endemic goiter. The results show differences in favor of the non-goiter areas. In Sicily, for example, the proportion of children with below-normal cognitive scores was 3% in areas with sufficient iodine, 18.5% in areas where iodine was inadequate, and 19.3% where iodine was inadequate and cretinism was endemic. Studies in Indonesia and Spain have documented similar effects on children in areas with insufficient iodine.

Fortification of school rations is the most efficient and effective route to alleviating micronutrient deficiencies in schoolchildren where SFPs are in operation. In South Africa, soup fortified with iron and vitamin C was provided to 350 schools in an area of low socio-economic development on the Cape Peninsula. Results showed that initially 12% of six to seven year old and 20% of 8 to 12 year old children had low weight-for-age, and 49% and 31% had low serum ferritin respectively. At follow-up, after 15 weeks of intervention, iron status improved significantly; falling from 49% to 28% in 6 to 7 year old children and 31% to 21% in 8 to 12 year old children.

A relatively new breakfast program in Peru, which includes an iron-fortified ration, was evaluated for its short-term impact on diet, amongst other factors. The program significantly increased dietary intakes of energy by 25%, protein by 28% and iron by 46%. A case-control study of the impact of providing heme-fortified cookies to school children in Chile found higher concentrations of hemoglobin among children receiving the fortified cookies through the school lunch program.

The impact was most significant among children with greater demands for iron such as post-menarchial girls and pubertal boys. Schools that depend on the community to organize and implement SFPs offer certain advantages. These advantages include: increasing the contact, and hence communication, between parents and teachers, officials and others; giving parents the opportunity to become more aware of what goes on at schools; and serving to raise the value of education/the school for parents and the whole community. For example, school canteens are viewed as an important feature of education policy in Morocco.

Since 1978 WFP and the government have supported school feeding. The programs have strong government and community support and are viewed as part of a necessary package of inputs for improving education. The feeding program is credited with helping to maintain high enrollment and attendance and encouraging community participation in education. School cooperatives support the school canteens and parents associations assist with the transportation of food aid.

The research and program literature on SFPs shows the potential that school feeding has to contribute to improving education. These focus on the most critical aspects of school feeding programming including targeting, cost and financing issues, ration composition and meal delivery, program implementation, and monitoring and evaluation, and on the integration of feeding with other interventions that address the nutrition and health needs of schoolchildren.

School feeding programs are highly visible and as a result often have a significant political dimension, particularly since they can represent a considerable income transfer. This reality should not inhibit establishing a policy and objectives that will take advantage of the substantial potential for improving the impact of SFPs on education.

Develop targeting criteria and mechanisms that concentrate program resources on high risk children and communities. There is a built-in tendency toward universal coverage - providing meals for all schoolchildren - since all children in school throughout *the day will require food. Furthermore, program coverage and targeting is always subject to a series of political, logistical, technical and informational constraints.*

In view of the fact that resources are finite, particularly in the poorest countries, and that providing food is expensive, targeting is a critical element of any effort to improve the impact of a SFP on education. Targeting is essential if the program is to reach families and communities that lack the resources to adequately provide for their school-age children or those that need to be motivated to enroll their children in school and to have them attend more regularly.

The cost of school feeding programs is a major issue for both governments and donors. Feeding programs of any kind are expensive. Financing may include international assistance, but in all cases available public resources, or the potential to draw on them, are required. Cost alone can indicate little about the value of a SFP but, unfortunately, cost-effectiveness analyses, which assess costs relative to impact on nutrition and education outcomes are for the most part unavailable.

Conditions in the education sector, such as levels of school enrollment, attendance, and performance, the availability of infrastructure and the capacity to implement different kinds of SFPs also need to be assessed. Information is also required on the community's perceptions and capacity to participate in school feeding programs.

Once school feeding programs are in place, altering them can meet strong resistance, however, a range of new experiences is now available that has the potential to alleviate some of the common obstacles to efficient and effective programming. Where a school feeding program already exists, a wealth of information is readily accessible; a critical step towards a better program is to thoroughly analyze this on-going experience.

Develop monitoring systems that focus on program processes, that is, how a program is functioning, and institute an evaluation system to assess the impact of the program on specific outcomes. The need to monitor and evaluate programs is not unique to SFPs, but this recommendation is critical to increasing the impact of SFPs. Despite decades of experience there is a dearth of concrete information on the functioning and effectiveness of school feeding programs.

Integrate feeding programs with other interventions that address the primary nutrition and health problems of the school-age population. The past decade has shown the added value of integrating other nutrition and health interventions with feeding. Specifically recommended are deworming, micronutrient fortification or supplementation, and health nutrition and hygiene education.

Although many SFPs have been conceived out of ideological, political and economic pressures, the prejudices of international or national personnel, or even commercial or other non-objective influences, the first step toward an effective program is to build programs on sound and transparent objectives. Since SFPs are highly visible and can offer a significant income transfer to families they will always be inherently political.

To avoid the use of programs for political purposes, information on programs - especially, who the program is for and why and targeting measures—must be made readily available to the public. Policy development and setting the objectives of school feeding provides the framework for implementing all the other recommendations aimed at improving the contribution that a SFP can make to education and better health and nutrition.

The process of policy development calls for compiling information on: what 'food-related' and education-related problems exist in the school-age population which could be addressed by school feeding; where, geographically, the problems are located; and which school feeding options are available, or could be developed, for addressing these problems.

Analyzing the nutrition and health situation of school-age children has become a way to engage governments in the problems of this age group. The appropriate method of collecting information will vary by needs, circumstances and resources. World Food Program has supported SFPs in the Gambia since 1971, providing a ration comprised of rice, wheat flour, canned meat, oil, and sugar.

The program has served on-site meals for about 92% of primary school children but resources for the program have been diminishing as enrollments have increased. Program administrators have diluted rations in lieu of targeting to particular regions or schools, maintaining 92% coverage. An effort was made to produce local foods in school gardens as a way to increase supplies, however, these efforts have not been wholly successful.

If the SFP is intended to motivate families to enroll children in school and to ensure more regular attendance, the target group is families whose children are not in school or who are frequently absent. Mechanisms and criteria for SFP targeting are similar in many cases to those used for other social programs: economic, geographic, and nutrition status. In addition, specific education criteria such as overall enrollment, female enrollment, absenteeism, or student performance would also be included under some circumstances.

In general it appears that SFP targeting is best done at the level of the school, or based on some other criteria - e.g., location - rather than on individual selection. The coverage of SFPs will depend on how many resources are available for programs and on the size of the problem that the program is intended to address. Economic or household income targeting is the most difficult of the targeting mechanisms available to implement, since measuring income is not straightforward, particularly where in-kind contributions to family income are substantial.

Community leaders, teachers, local government entities or voluntary organizations can participate in identifying the poorest households, but this requires clear criteria that are transparent and not based on political favoritism. If economic targeting is already in place for other programs, the school program could build on it, however, singling out individual children in a classroom or school for a feeding program or for a reduced price can be stigmatizing and socially and politically unacceptable.

School feeding programming, particularly that supported by the WFP, has recently concentrated on addressing the need to encourage female enrollment and continuation in both primary and secondary school.

Toward this end programs are not only targeted at specific regions within countries where female participation in school is a problem, but the ration provided to girls may be of higher nutritional and caloric content to serve as an even greater incentive for girls to attend and stay in school. In some cases the continuation of WFP-assisted programs is contingent on a certain proportion of girls participating in the program.

In Pakistan a WFP-assisted program provides an income transfer of one or two tins of oil to families whose girls attend school for 20 days a month. In participating schools enrollment increased by 76% compared to 14% in the province. Attendance also increased from 76 to 93% in participating schools. In Bhutan, a similar program that provides an additional meal for girls has increased attendance in lower grades and newer schools. School enrollment has not changed since demand for school already outstrips supply.

In Niger, where school enrollment is one of the lowest in the world, a WFP-assisted program is providing, in some areas, the equivalent of the total daily recommended food intake in three meals a day, as well as a take-home ration to attract nomadic girls to school. Evidence shows that when school canteens have been closed immediate and high absenteeism follows and children are withdrawn from school. Often the school year cannot start in some nomadic areas until the food stocks have arrived.

SFPs, by virtue of the fact that they include food, are expensive. Beyond the costs of the food itself, the costs associated with food management, logistics and control can represent a significant financial burden for governments. On-site feeding is costly as it requires daily preparation and delivery of food, but is also a model that can invite, or require, community participation. In response to the difficulties of on-site feeding and a new focus on delivering an appropriately-timed and high quality, consistent ration, some countries are developing program models that include less costly commodities and more efficient systems for delivery to schools.

Programs that make good use of the education infrastructure for delivery and logistics will be most efficient. The very fact that SFPs do not require, for the most part, additional infrastructure means that they can be less costly than other types of feeding programs which distribute benefits to groups that are not in one location. Programs that finance expensive kitchen equipment and supplies or build new infrastructure/ canteens, however, will significantly raise the costs and lower the relative cost-effectiveness of programs.

Some SFPs are intentionally designed as an income-transfer for families, especially those that are trying to help attract girls to schools; the benefit received by families from these programs must therefore surpass the costs of having their daughters away from home attending school. A comparison of the costs of SFPs is problematic; the number of feeding days varies, as does the quantity of the rations and their quality. In the early 1990s two sizable studies made some accurate comparisons of cross-country cost information by standardizing and controlling for some of these differences.

New Approaches of School Feeding

The new SFP in Indonesia is providing between US$0.10 and US$0.15 per ration per day to village schools via the village bank. The guidelines for the relatively small, locally made ration are that it should contain 300 kcal and about 5 grams of protein. It will be provided three times a week for nine months. The key to the Indonesian program is not only that it is a snack program, intended to be additional to rather than replacing a family meal, but that the food is integrated with other interventions - deworming, health and nutrition education and water and sanitation.

In South Africa, a national school breakfast program takes a similar approach with decentralized management, provision of funds for local food purchases and integrated interventions. The estimated cost of the ration, which will provide about 25% of the recommended daily allowance (RDA) for calories is about US$0.30 per child per day. An additional 10% per child per day is intended to cover local operating costs.

Bolivia's new USAID-assisted SFP is integrated with the educational reform underway in Bolivia. One objective of the reform is to increase parental involvement in education and the SFP is one mechanism for this. The municipalities will pay about US$1.60 per student per year and contribute to transportation costs of the donated foods from warehouses to schools. The total cost per child per year is estimated at US$4.00 for a snack program consisting of fortified bread and hot chocolate. The program will also integrate parasite treatment, health education and vision and hearing screening.

Financial Support of School Feeding Programme

Food aid is an important source of support for SFPs. There are high costs associated with transportation, warehouses and distribution; adequate storage facilities are required at every stage from port to the point of distribution. These costs are often borne by recipient governments. Management and distribution of food requires trained people to keep track of food inventories and their location, human resources may be as much of a constraint as cash and physical facilities.

Nonetheless, if the economic and financial costs are acceptable then the cost of these programs may not be prohibitive relative to the benefit provided. Drawing on the private sector for school feeding programming overcomes many of the difficulties of on-site preparation of meals, and may be one of the least costly ways to feed children in schools. The private sector in this case can be street vendors, local canteen or a large canteen company (in cities and more commercially sophisticated areas).

However, even these programs incur costs in monitoring and supervision, and the start-up costs for developing school meal alternatives and making arrangements with vendors can be substantial. Programs that utilize school canteens or street food vendors for school-based feeding programs may offer the most economical approach to school feeding. However, the technical and logistical implications, and hence costs in training and supplies to improve the provision of food through these sources are not insubstantial.

Certain food selections are particularly expensive;

foremost among these is milk, which is expensive per the number of calories, and nutrients it provides, and is perishable, which if figured in with the cost increases costs even further. UHT milk alternatives, which overcome the perishability issues, are particularly expensive to produce, especially in developing countries where the relevant technology is not widespread. Parent-teacher or other community associations can play a significant role in a SFP and ultimately assume some of the costs.

Where feasible, more refined targeting mechanisms that maximize the participation of the most needy populations improve the efficiency of programs. Ultimately this can mean charging fees to students who can afford them for participation in the program. Food transfer programs cannot be considered 'sustainable' in the same way as, for example, a revolving credit program, which ultimately pays for itself. A continual input of resources is required in order to provide food for school children. From the perspective of the individual beneficiary, the sustainable aspect of the program is likely to be the lasting impact on behavior changes brought about through education or other interventions that are part of the program.

School meals provided early in the school day to alleviate hunger before or while classes are in session should help to improve attention, concentration, and achievement among children. Historically, and even now, political and social objectives dominate in school feeding programming. School meals were viewed, and in many cases still are, as a means for a school child to receive a large meal in the middle of the day, which typically coincides with local dietary practices. These programs served, and continue to serve, not only as nutrition programs, but perhaps more as social welfare programs that provide a substantial economic benefit to the family since the child will not eat at mid-day from the family pot.

Nonetheless, the nutritional quality and quantity of a ration should always be assessed as well as the effects of the timing of ration delivery. Other factors such as local food habits, logistical considerations, food availability, and cost will also influence the selection of the ration. General ration guidelines that can be applied almost universally are:

— *A school snack or meal usually provides from one-third to one-half of the recommended daily allowance for energy and protein for the school-age group targeted by the program. A substantial ration is recommended to ensure overcompensating in order that parents don't withdraw more food at home than the child receives at school. Programs which include older children, particularly adolescents, in the target group will require larger rations to meet the increased nutritional needs during this period.*

— *Rations that fill the actual micronutrient gaps in the diets of school-age children are higher in nutritional quality and can be expected to have greater impacts on learning. Ensuring that the appropriate level of micronutrients is included in the school ration may require more than selecting the appropriate mix of foods. Fortification may be an option if the size of the ration is relatively small, where the ration itself, or a component like flour, is centrally processed, or where the foods to be used do not contain a high level of the most critical micronutrients.*

— *Fresh milk, although it appears to be nutritious and convenient, is not recommended as it is usually an expensive source of calories and is perishable and subject to contamination.*

— *A meal or snack provided early in the school day will eliminate hunger so that children are more attentive in class.*

WFP-assisted programs offer the option of using fortified blended foods such as corn-soy blend or wheat-soy blend. These foods provide at least two-thirds of the daily micronutrient requirements of young children. Local alternative programs such as the snack programs in the Dominican Republic and Peru offer another approach to providing a fortified ration. In the Dominican Republic the corn meal used in the production of the cookies and muffins for the SFP is fortified with 100% of the iron requirement for young children. All producers must purchase and use this corn meal in the production of the school ration.

Similarly in Peru, one requirement in selecting producers of the grain product for the SFP was that the product contains at least two-thirds of the daily requirement for iron and vitamin A. In many cases the current emphasis on the timing of meals - providing the school meal early in the day to maximize the impact of the program on educational objectives- involves a significant change from current practice. Furthermore, given the conditions for meal preparation in many developing countries - e.g., the need to utilize volunteers, long distances to fetch water and fuel for cooking, slow cooking facilities - the successful preparation and provision of meals to children early in the day is not easy.

New program approaches have recently been developed and tested to overcome some of the technical and logistical obstacles associated with SFPs that countries might consider in developing new and modifying on-going programs:

Use of snack foods: Providing a snack as opposed to what may be a more traditional school meal (school lunch) will significantly cut the preparation time. In Indonesia, for example, a new program will provide from 10 to 15 US cents per ration for the local production of a snack food with 300 kcal and 5 grams of protein. The intent of this program is specifically to avoid industrially produced snack foods, since another objective is to increase local food production, however, the emphasis is equally on the delivery of an appropriately-timed snack.

The basic foods to be used are tubers (cassava sweet potato, taro), cereals (rice, corn), fruits, and vegetables. Snack foods also avoid the problem of substitution of the school meal for one of the family meals; this is preferable from a nutritional perspective since the school meal will be additional to the normal diet.

Products with quicker cooking times: Blended foods and cereal flours can be prepared much more quickly than unmilled whole grains. In Kenya, for example, a long-running program that provided a school lunch to children involved more than 4 hours of preparation time.

Monetization: Monetization is the sale of donated foods in the general market so that the central government can give the proceeds to school systems for feeding programs; the school systems then purchase the food in their local communities. This practice obviates the need to transport large quantities of food around countries, which in many cases is a severe obstacle to implementing consistent and effective programs. It also can increase the choice of food commodities that can be used in the feeding program. This practice is becoming increasingly popular. Although it generates income for the local economy, putting donated food in the market can depress indigenous food production and increase the risk of mismanagement and corruption. Issues of food preparation also need to be addressed.

The private sector: The off-site prepared meal/snack program addresses many of the technical and logistical concerns of SFPs. Programs in Peru and the Dominican Republic are examples of the private sector approach to school meals. In both cases the meal provided is a snack or breakfast which is itself a break from the traditional school lunch. Utilizing private enterprises to prepare and deliver the snack foods to schools facilitates the provision of the ration early in the day as well as ensuring a consistent and high quality ration while taking a minimal time away from learning. One problem with these programs can be the monotony of the ration.

The informal private sector/street vendors: Enlisting the support of local street vendors to provide better quality school meals to children is an option to consider. In Lesotho, for example, former local vendors who successfully bid to provide the privatized service run school canteens. In Nigeria, state and local governments train and license vendors who sell to schoolchildren. In other cases school principals exercise their authority locally and choose the vendors to serve their schools. A major concern that must be addressed in using this

5

Health Promoting Schools

Children are also future parents. There is evidence that children with appropriate knowledge and motivation can be effective motivators of change in the home. As well as assisting with the construction, maintenance and cleaning of facilities in the school environment, studies reveal that promoting latrine construction through school children can be a successful medium for promoting construction in the wider community.

Tobacco Use Prevention

Tobacco use prevention deserves increased attention and support Schools, communities and nations urgently need to increase efforts to prevent tobacco use, especially among young people. WHO estimates that one out of two young people who start smoking and continue smoking throughout their lives will ultimately be killed by a tobacco-related illness.

Tobacco is a known or probable cause of about 25 diseases. The sheer scale of its impact on global disease burden is still not fully appreciated. It is well known that tobacco is the most important cause of lung cancer, for example; less well know is the fact that it kills even more people through other diseases, including cancers at other sites, heart disease, stroke, emphysema and other chronic lung diseases.

Smokeless tobacco causes oral cancer, especially in the lip, tongue, mouth and throat area, and is associated with cancer in the digestive system. The annual mortality from tobacco chewing in South Asia alone may well be above 50,000 deaths a year. Breathing Environmental Tobacco Smoke (ETS) (i.e. side-stream and exhaled smoke from cigarettes, cigars and pipes) causes serious health problems.(1) ETS can aggravate allergies and increase the severity of symptoms in children and adolescents with asthma and heart disease; it is also associated with lung cancer because ETS contains essentially the same cancer-causing substances and toxic agents that are inhaled by the smoker.

If parents use tobacco, children can suffer health consequences. Maternal smoking is associated with a higher risk of miscarriage, lower birth weight of babies and inhibited child development. Parental smoking is also a factor in Sudden Infant Death Syndrome (SIDS) and is associated with higher rates of respiratory illnesses, including bronchitis, colds and pneumonia in their children.

Most people who use tobacco were influenced to start during their school-age years. The majority of tobacco users begin while in their teenage years or earlier. In many countries, tobacco use is rising among young people, while the age of tobacco use initiation is descending. In Latin American countries, 75% or more of smoking initiation occurs between the ages of 14 and 17.

We know what influences young people to use tobacco Complex and inter-related factors influence children's and adolescents' use of tobacco. First and foremost, young people interpret smoking as a sign of independence -an image they see in adults who smoke and one which is skillfully created by tobacco advertising. Adults who smoke, such as family members, film stars and sports heroes strongly influence children, and especially adolescents. In many countries, large numbers of teachers, medical professionals, politicians and government officials use tobacco.

Tobacco advertising plays a key role in encouraging young people to smoke. In countries around the world, billions of dollars are being spent on sophisticated tobacco advertising and promotions, portraying tobacco use as "fun", "glamorous", "mature", "modern" and "Western". At school, social relations influence the way young people live, their norms and values. Research suggests that young people are most at risk for starting tobacco use when they make the transition from primary to secondary school and when they come in contact with older students who use tobacco.

In the transition from primary school to secondary school (and from childhood to adolescence) the need to be part of a group often becomes paramount. Differences in image and lifestyle to distinguish one group from another; this can include the use of tobacco. Group norms can play a significant role in pressuring young people to use tobacco; vulnerability to this pressure may be greater in young people with poor relationships, low self-esteem, boredom and social disadvantage.

Older students are role models for younger students; their tobacco use encourages younger students to believe that tobacco is part of a mature image. Group members and older students who do not use tobacco, and who support the decisions of others to avoid its use, play an important role in preventing the initiation of tobacco use among young people.

Prevention is a critically important strategy for reducing tobacco use among young people. Young people tend to underestimate how addictive nicotine is:

- *The younger people are when they start smoking cigarettes, the more likely they are to become strongly addicted to nicotine.*
- *Even trying cigarettes is dangerous. One-third to one-half of adolescents who experiment with cigarettes go on to become regular smokers. One study found that among those who experimented with cigarettes, about one-half had become regular smokers within one year.*
- *Young people also tend to underestimate how difficult it is to stop using tobacco:*
- *Although intentions to quit and quit attempts are common among teenagers, only small numbers of teenagers actually stop.*
- *Studies in the United States have found that about 75% of young smokers considered themselves addicted; about 66% of adolescent smokers indicated that they wanted to quit; and about 70% said that*

would not have started if they could choose again.

— *People who start using tobacco early have more difficulty quitting, are more likely to become heavy smokers and are more likely to develop a smoking-related disease.*

Programmes that prevent the initiation of tobacco use among school-age children and adolescents are strategically important because of tobacco's impact on health and education. As the age at which young people initiate tobacco use decreases, an increased proportion of these people will eventually develop tobacco-related diseases, raising the already burdensome costs of treatment for these diseases.

Studies carried out in many countries show that if young people do not begin to use tobacco before the age of 20, they are unlikely to start smoking as adults. Preventing tobacco use among young people helps prevent long-term health problems and premature death, and promotes optimal health. Preventing tobacco use among school students decreases school days missed because of respiratory illnesses.

Cessation can be an important element of a prevention/reduction strategy. The seemingly discouraging results of tobacco use cessation programmes have reinforced the opinion that more systematic attention must be given to policies and programmes that prevent individuals from starting to use tobacco. However, successful cessation efforts can support prevention efforts and yield substantial health benefits for young and adult tobacco users, as well as for people who would otherwise be exposed to their smoke. o Health promotion efforts to persuade young people not to use tobacco are likely to be more successful when they also increase attention to helping tobacco users quit.

One year after quitting, the risk of coronary heart disease decreases by 50% and within 15 years, the risk approaches that of a long-time non-smoker. The relative risk of developing lung cancer, chronic obstructive lung diseases and stroke also decreases, but more slowly. Cessation benefits health, no matter at what age one quits smoking; it also helps reduce the existence of Environmental Tobacco Smoke, which is harmful to non-smokers as well as smokers.

Tobacco use prevention is among the most cost-effective of health promotion interventions. Tobacco use, a major drain on the world's financial resources, has been labeled a major threat to sustainable and equitable development. Tobacco products cause a loss to the world economy that is so great that a conservative estimate ranks it as an amount that exceeds total current health expenditures in all developing countries combined. A World Bank study estimated that the use of tobacco results in a global net loss of US$200 billion per year, with half of these losses occurring in developing countries.

The World Bank also estimated that smoking prevention is among the most cost-effective of all health interventions. The same study cited school health programmes that provide school health services and health education as among the most cost-effective of the public health interventions compared. Tobacco use prevention programmes can be a good entry point for the development of Health-Promoting Schools

Experience has shown that important health issues

can serve as effective entry points for the development of Health-Promoting Schools. Schools are vital partners for achieving WHO's vision of "Growing Up Tobacco Free" Schools have organizational potential and access to a large number of children, adolescents and adults who can help make WHO's vision of "Growing Up Tobacco Free" a reality. Schools can be vital partners to WHO and other relevant organizations that share these characteristics:

— *The belief that every child has the right to grow up without tobacco and without the pressures to use tobacco that emanate from a variety of sources in many schools, communities and nations.*

— *The determination to help change the environment so that non-smoking is considered normal social behaviour and the choice not to smoke is the easier choice.*

— *The willingness to call upon and work concertedly with governments and other sectors to implement "A Ten Point Programme for Successful Tobacco Control"*

School-based prevention programmes that identify the social influences prompting youth to smoke and that teach skills to resist these influences have demonstrated consistent and significant reductions or delays in adolescent smoking. These programmes usually target youth in their early teenage years, when smoking experimentation and initiation is most common. Effects of these prevention programmes dissipate with time, but can be enhanced with booster sessions or further application of the programme.

The difference in smoking rates or initiation

between treatment and non-treatment student groups ranges from 25% to 60% and persists from one to four years. Effectiveness of school-based programmes appears to be strengthened by community-wide programmes that involve parents, school policies, mass media and youth access, and mobilize community organizations. The tendency for positive effects to dissipate over time has been particularly evident in school-based intervention studies that include little or no emphasis on booster sessions, few (if any) community-wide activities or policy interventions, or few (if any) mass-media-based components.

A school-based prevention programme on its own has limitations in impact and scope. Any effort to prevent adolescent tobacco initiation or dependence must address the social context for tobacco use. Initial studies suggest that the combination of school and community prevention programmes can enhance the impact of the school-based programme by providing a complementary, longer-term and multi-pronged approach.

Given the number of studies, the variability in programme format and scope, the various communities and subcultures in which these studies were implemented and the potential threats to internal and external validity in school-based research, the consistency in overall reductions in smoking prevalence across all these studies is remarkable.

The "interactive" nature of the prevention programme was the distinguishing feature for successful programmes regardless of who lead the programme. What appears to matter most is whether the leader can facilitate the necessary group interactions. A meta-

analysis of 90 school-based tobacco use prevention programmes designed to develop skills to use in resisting social-influence indicated that tobacco use was 4.5% lower among students in programmes that focussed on social influence than among control groups.

The most effective programmes were delivered to 6 th grade students, used booster sessions, concentrated the programme in a short time period and used peers to present the programmes. Furthermore, informal learning experiences in school can significantly influence students' attitudes and behaviours. Schools can place fragmented and ad hoc information on tobacco use from mass media, peers and relevant adults into a more comprehensive framework.

Over a period of time, schools can approach students in a systematic, process-oriented way. Schools can address various tobacco use topics and their links with risk-taking behaviours (that involve other drugs, alcohol and illicit drugs) relevant to particular age groups. Moreover, schools can provide a planned and sequenced curriculum that systematically discusses different attitudes and develops skills in students at various ages.

When schools set up school-wide activities, based upon multiple strategies and involving parents and community members, the whole school population can benefit from tobacco use prevention. Combining school interventions with community action and support enhances the effects of the interventions.

Tobacco use prevention can be an entry point for schools that want to build their capacity to plan and implement a wide range of health promotion efforts.

The first step is to recognize tobacco use prevention as a priority for both education and health. The next step is to plan interventions: determine which strategies will have the most significant influence on conditions and behaviours related to tobacco use and how to integrate such interventions with other health promotion efforts for maximum results.

Policies to protect children from tobacco

A School Health Team is a group of people working together to maintain and promote the health of all people who are working and learning at school. Policies to protect children from tobacco can be passed in many forms and at many different levels of government (e.g., local, provincial, national and international). Policies may be passed most easily as regulations in some places and as legislation in others.

In most countries, nongovernmental organizations (NGOs) play a critical role in promoting passage of tobacco prevention laws. National and local policies and commitments can maximize the success of local efforts to prevent and reduce tobacco use through schools. Schools can help to foster supportive policies. Children do not simply "choose" to smoke. They are greatly influenced by their environment.

Their environments influence their "choices" and public policies influence their environments. Children are much more likely to smoke if they are surrounded by attractive tobacco advertising and promotion; if their favourite sport is sponsored by a tobacco company; if their film idols smoke in the movies; if they see people smoking all around them; and if tobacco products are cheap and readily available.

Without sound public policies, the billions of dollars tobacco companies spend promoting their products and creating a "pro-tobacco" environment for children can overwhelm the prevention efforts of parents and schools. Strong public policies help level the playing field and give children a real chance to grow up tobacco-free.

Policy experts agree that a combination of the policies described below should significantly reduce tobacco use by youth, provided they are sustained over time, strictly enforced and adequately funded. Although benefits will be realised through the implementation of even one of these policies, a comprehensive approach works best.

For real progress to be made, all of the recommended policies need to be implemented. Tobacco companies, denied one approach to marketing or selling tobacco products to children, will attempt to use any other methods that are not prohibited. Higher tobacco taxation Studies consistently show that tobacco use among children is more sensitive to price increases than tobacco use among adults.

In the United States, for example, youth are about three times more likely than adults to quit smoking, or not to start smoking, in response to a tobacco price increase. Increasing the price puts a higher barrier between youth and easy access. Thus tobacco tax increases are good health policy and good fiscal policy. Cheap cigarettes are not a social benefit: they encourage more smoking, causing higher health care costs and more death and disease.

Another way to make cheap cigarettes less accessible to young people would be to legislate against single sales of cigarettes as well as half-size cigarette packages, known in some countries as "kiddie packs". In many countries, governments earn substantial tax revenue from illegal sales of tobacco products to minors, but often put only a small percentage back into prevention programmes for young people.

It is highly appropriate that a portion of funds raised by tobacco taxes fund programs to protect children and reduce tobacco use. This funding approach has been used in Australia, the United States, Canada and other countries; it is effective and politically popular. Advertising affects young people's perceptions of the pervasiveness, image and functions of smoking. Studies have shown that in some countries tobacco advertising is twice as influential as peer pressure in encouraging children to smoke.

Children are more likely to buy the most heavily advertised brands of cigarettes. Because tobacco advertising is inherently misleading, public policies should prohibit all tobacco advertising and promotions, including free samples and other give-aways, sale of non-tobacco products that carry a tobacco brand name, point of sale advertising and tobacco company sponsorship of sporting and cultural events.

Countries that have adopted bans on tobacco advertising as part of a comprehensive tobacco control programme have seen significant declines in tobacco consumption. In many countries, tobacco products are routinely sold to children (although sales of other addictive, lethal drugs to children are not tolerated). A minimum age of 18 or older should be established for tobacco sales.

All tobacco retailers should be licensed and their license should be contingent on obeying the law. A graduated schedule of civil penalties ranging from a warning to license revocation should be established. Enforcement is critically important! If these laws are not enforced, they will not be obeyed. Enforcement funds may be raised from licensing fees and penalties, so these measures can be self-supporting. To eliminate possibilities of unsupervised sales of tobacco products, vending machine sales should be prohibited.

Protection from environmental tobacco smoke

Smoking should be legally prohibited in public places, especially where children may be present. Environmental Tobacco Smoke (ETS) is known to be harmful, especially to children. If public places become smoke-free, then young people will have far fewer places to light up, which could go a long way in reducing smoking. Finally, children who grow up seeing smoking permitted all around them will wrongly conclude that smoke must not be very harmful, and that it is socially acceptable to smoke.

The awareness and commitment of parents are central to the success of efforts to prevent and reduce tobacco use through schools. Parents influence their children's health directly by providing a smoking or non-smoking home environment, they convey norms and serve as role models. Ensuring that parents recognize and understand the consequences of tobacco use can help bring about support and action.

Involve parents and family members to reinforce on-going school efforts to influence behaviours and the conditions that reduce and prevent tobacco use and exposure to environmental tobacco smoke. Mobilize parental support through special meetings at school, focussed on issues such as preventing tobacco use at every grade level, problems faced by children who are about to move from primary to secondary school and especially decisions to use tobacco.

Goals and Objectives

Using the information gathered in the situation analysis, the School Health Team, in collaboration with the Community Advisory Committee, is ready to develop a vision for change and an action plan. This provides a basis for formulating goals and objectives for health promotion and tobacco use prevention interventions.

Goals make clear what the programme should achieve and describe in broad terms what the programme will do. Tobacco-related goals of a Health-Promoting School aim to:

— *prevent the initiation of tobacco use*

— *reduce the proportion of individuals who use tobacco*

— *prevent exposure to environmental tobacco smoke*

Goals are then broken down into specific outcome and process objectives so that everyone clearly understands what needs to be done, when and why. In measurable terms, what the interventions will achieve in terms of knowledge, attitudes, beliefs, skills, behaviours and conditions related to tobacco use and interventions. Examples of outcome objectives of comprehensive tobacco use prevention interventions include:

- *a specified reduction, each year, in the proportion of children who initiate tobacco use*
- *a specified reduction, each year, in the proportion of children who use tobacco regularly*
- *a specified change in knowledge, attitudes and skills needed to avoid tobacco use and create tobacco-free conditions*
- *delay in the age when children start tobacco use*

A Health-Promoting School strives to use the school's full organisational capacity to improve the health of students, school personnel, families and community members. Such a school offers many opportunities to promote tobacco use prevention as an essential element in maintaining health.

Tobacco use prevention interventions can serve as an entry point for developing or enhancing policies, planning groups and various components that serve as a framework for a Health-Promoting School. These components include, but are not limited to:

- *school health education*
- *healthy school environment*
- *school health services*
- *school/community projects and outreach*
- *health promotion for school staff*
- *school safety*
- *physical exercise, recreation and sport*
- *counselling and social support.*

Effectiveness of interventions integrated into each of these components depends on the extent to which they are supported by people, policies and trained staff and also how successfully the components combine with other health promotion efforts to complement and reinforce one another. Not every school will have the resources to integrate tobacco use interventions into all of the components at one time.

Therefore, each school has to establish its own priorities, in collaboration with all parties concerned, to decide how thoroughly the components will be addressed. A Health-Promoting School enables students, parents, teachers and community members to work together to make such decisions. It is better to start with small changes as early as possible than to wait until resources become available to address all of these components at once.

The primary goals of school health education are to help individuals adopt behaviours and create conditions that are conducive to health. The clear and precise delineation of behaviours and conditions that are to be influenced is essential for the development of effective school health education efforts. Examples of behaviours and conditions commonly addressed to prevent or reduce tobacco use include:

- *resisting peer pressure to smoke cigarettes*
- *trying cigarette smoking for the first time*
- *smoking a whole cigarette*
- *smoking cigarettes on a regular basis*
- *smoking cigarettes on the school property*
- *attempting to quit cigarette smoking*

— *chewing tobacco*

— *creating a tobacco-free school policy*

— *creating tobacco-free public areas*

Some programmes to prevent tobacco use have been limited to providing factual information about the harmful effects of tobacco use. Other programmes have attempted to induce fear in young persons about the consequences of use. These strategies alone do not prevent tobacco use, however; they may stimulate curiosity about tobacco use and prompt some students to believe that the health hazards of tobacco use are exaggerated.

In a Health-Promoting School, education to prevent tobacco use is designed to help students acquire the knowledge, attitudes, beliefs and skills they need to make informed decisions, practice healthy behaviours and create conditions conducive to health. Interventions should help students understand that tobacco use can result in death and disease, such as heart disease and cancer; and that it has immediate effects such as decreased stamina, stained teeth, foul-smelling breath and clothes, exacerbation of asthma and ostracism by non-smoking peers.

Interventions should use educational techniques to decrease the social acceptability of tobacco use, highlight existing anti-tobacco norms and help students understand that most adolescents do not smoke. Interventions should help students understand that many adolescents use tobacco because they believe it will help them be accepted by peers, appear mature or cope with stress. Interventions should help students develop other, more positive means to attain such goals.

Interventions should help students develop skills in recognising and refusing tobacco promotion messages from the tobacco industry, the media, adults and peers. Behavioural skills for resisting social influences that promote tobacco use. Interventions should help students develop refusal skills through direct instruction, modelling, role playing, rehearsal and reinforcement; and should coach them to help others develop refusal skills.

Interventions should help students develop the skills to make healthy decisions, solve problems, think creatively and critically, communicate effectively, maintain positive relationships, cope with emotions and stress and develop an adequate sense of empathy and self awareness in order to avoid tobacco use and other health risk behaviours.

In a Health-Promoting School, school health education systematically addresses these and other relevant factors at developmentally appropriate ages. Specific examples of knowledge, attitudes and skills that might be addressed at early and late, primary and secondary school levels are described below.

School health education needs to offer a planned, sequential course of instruction from the primary level through the secondary level, addressing the physical, mental and social dimensions of health. It can be taught as a specific subject, integrated into other subjects or a combination of both approaches. It can also be included in extracurricular activities.

Because most young people start using tobacco as adolescents, more intensive instructional programmes should be provided for these age groups. Particularly important is the transition from primary to secondary school when new students have to learn to get along with a wider group of peers and come in contact with older students who may use tobacco.

For these reasons, interventions need to be especially intensive in early secondary school: for instance, through a minimum of five lessons upon entrance to secondary school followed by booster sessions in the following years. Annual preventive education, such as booster sessions, can reinforce the educational interventions in secondary school. Without continued reinforcement (follow-up), success in preventing tobacco use can dissipate over time.

Health education to prevent tobacco use will enhance the overall framework of a Health-Promoting School if it is integrated into other school health components, such as physical activity and health promotion for staff. Furthermore, it should be combined with efforts that address other health issues, such as use of alcohol and other substances, life skills and injury prevention, so that the learning experiences will complement and reinforce one another. Link these issues by integrating them into a school health education curriculum and coordinating the simultaneous or sequential presentation of related topics in different classes.

Tobacco use prevention and other relevant topics can also be linked through co-teaching, sharing teaching resources, referring students to related lessons and involving students from different classes in group activities. Curricula for tobacco use prevention and other health-related issues may be available through governmental and non-governmental agencies and organizations, universities or teachers' unions.

Teachers and students themselves may also create supplemental materials specific to the local situation. Some educational interventions are more effective than others in influencing certain factors. Select an educational method based on how appropriate that method is to influence the factors, such as knowledge, attitudes and skills associated with tobacco use and conditions that contribute to the initiation, maintenance and cessation of tobacco use.

When developing school policy and programmes, make efforts to involve students. Students can play an important role in deciding on a policy and in developing and implemening interventions. Students can also contribute to carrying out the interventions by modelling social skills and leading role rehearsals. Peer leaders can help counteract social pressures that encourage youth to use tobacco, especially if they receive training so that they accurately present skills and information.

School and community environments play a significant role in determining whether interventions to prevent and reduce tobacco use will be effective and sustainable. To create an environment that supports health education and tobacco use prevention, a Health-Promoting School must consider its policies and management practices.

Supportive school policies, brief documents that promote a clear set of school norms regarding health and tobacco use, guide schools in planning, implementing and evaluating efforts to promote health and prevent tobacco use. They incorporate input from all relevant members of the school community: students, teachers, parents, staff, administrators, health service providers and counsellors.

School policies need to meet national and local rules and should be adapted to the health concerns and practices of different ethnic and cultural groups represented. Policies also need to support collaboration and coordination among the health, education and economic sectors, and the school and community.

Students, teachers and other school personnel are not allowed to use tobacco except in one room or area on the school property. A tobacco-free school: tobacco use is not allowed within the school premises, on the schoolyard and in the immediate surroundings. To ensure broad support for school policies on tobacco, the School Health Team, Community Advisory Committee, representatives of relevant groups (students, parents, school staff and their unions) and school board members should participate in developing and implementing the policy.

A Health-Promoting School provides an ambience that respects the individual and fosters confidence in healthy choices and healthy lifestyles. Aspects of a healthy psycho-social environment to be integrated into a Health-Promoting School: Support for not using tobacco and cessation: The psycho-social environment should support health-conducive perceptions and actions of all who learn, work and play in the school. It should be consistent with other health-promoting interventions in the school and the classroom.

For instance, the friendliness and support of school staff as well as the community members involved in the projects can contribute encouragement and psycho-social support for those who are trying to quit using tobacco. One aspect of the school's psycho-social environment is the important role that teachers play as adult role models and as mentors. For instance, teachers can set an example and encourage students to follow a healthy way of life by not using tobacco.

Young people influence each other. Students can provide positive reinforcement to their peers by showing that tobacco use is not an essential element to being accepted by peers. This requires students to be provided with time and opportunities to stimulate socialization without social pressure to use tobacco. School health services help foster health and well-being as well as prevent, reduce, monitor or treat important health problems or conditions.

In Health-Promoting Schools, health services work in partnership with and are provided for students, school personnel, families and community members. They are coordinated with other services and tobacco use prevention activities at school and in the community. They use specialists to provide advice and support for health promotion and tobacco use prevention. Schools and communities need to consider what preventive and treatment services are necessary for prevention and cessation (e.g. cessation programmes, counselling) and how these can best be provided.

Effective coordination avoids duplicating services. Give special attention to ensuring that services are easily accessible for students and school personnel. Health service providers know the health consequences of tobacco use. Complementary community-wide strategies can strengthen education interventions. Health-Promoting Schools provide a valuable link to parents and community members who can support and encourage children to make choices that promote health. Schools, families and the community should work together to improve health and prevent tobacco use within the community.

In a Health-Promoting School, personnel, community members and families can participate together in planning and implementing tobacco-free activities that strengthen community spirit and health. Tobacco use prevention activities provide excellent opportunities to undertake school/community projects that can affect the health status of the entire community. These projects give students a chance to become actively involved in learning how to prevent tobacco use.

Family involvement

The family provides a setting where students can understand, practice and share what they learn in the classroom about health and tobacco use. Potentially, families can support and reinforce tobacco use prevention and health promotion. Thus, it is essential for school staff and parents to work together in order to maximize the potential for prevention both at school and at home.

Students are most likely to adopt healthy lifestyle patterns if they receive consistent information and support through multiple channels; parents, peers, teachers, community members and the media. Therefore, a school trying to prevent students from starting to use tobacco needs to strengthen links and involve parents as much as possible. Parents, in turn, should feel that their school is open and receptive to their ideas and participation. Establish connections with parents during school health fairs, health-related workshops for parents, parent-teacher meetings or a parent's visit to relevant services at school or in the community.

The school can provide parents and family members with information, resources and skills related to tobacco use prevention in an effort to extend the school interventions into the students' homes. Involving parents in tobacco use prevention at the primary school level (for example through take-home activities and interventions at school) can discourage tobacco use in both students and their parents.

In addition to learning how to prevent and reduce tobacco use for themselves and their children, parents can contribute services or resources to the school and participate or lead community efforts that promote tobacco use prevention. Outreach to community and family members is especially important in places where a high percentage of young people do not attend school. School outreach to the community has the potential to reach those who have no direct contact with the school.

Role of Mass media

Many governments have established successful programs, using mass media to provide strong messages designed to counter the image of tobacco use as sexy, glamorous and normal. Equally important are school-based and community-based prevention programs. Research shows that coordinated mass media programs and education programs produce much better results than either approach by itself.

Mass media can attract attention to the issue of tobacco use and provide information on prevention activities. It can be used on a national and local scale as well as in classrooms for health promotion and tobacco use prevention. Mass media include well-known channels such as radio, television, signboards and written materials (newspapers, magazines, booklets, leaflets).

Calendars, comics, photo novels, posters and traditional communication forms, such as dance troupes, are also channels to communicate a message. Radio programmes, television shows, quiz programmes for schoolchildren and crossword puzzles in children's newspapers have been used to prevent children from initiating tobacco use.

Some materials can be distributed through more than one channel or can be used with different target groups: a teacher with a cassette recorder can play the same programme at the village well that is broadcast over radio or discussed in class. Multimedia approaches that combine face-to-face and mass channels are appropriate for tobacco use prevention because tobacco use is relevant to everybody (through smoking or environmental tobacco smoke); different channels are necessary for different phases in the learning process.

Tobacco company advertising is a pervasive and influential aspect of the media, especially when targeted at adolescents. Therefore, it is important to teach children to understand how advertising encourages tobacco use. If health-promoting organizations are involved in school and community prevention efforts, they can help inform students about manipulative advertising. Schools can also use special student projects (such as, encouraging students to work with media to design campaigns) to encourage the media to help prevent tobacco use and discourage tobacco promotion and advertising.

A Health-Promoting School does not limit its efforts to preventing tobacco use among students: it also emphasizes tobacco use prevention and cessation for employees, teachers, administrators and support staff. Counselling and courses can help the school staff quit using tobacco. As school personnel in most countries have little or no training and/or experience with tobacco cessation, training may be needed.

A Health-Promoting School strives to provide healthy working conditions for all staff: it is important to establish regulations on tobacco use on the school premises, within classrooms and other areas. As policies are developed, communicated them to students and employees, explaining the changes concerning tobacco use, the rationale behind them and when they come into effect. Offer support to employees to help them quit tobacco use.

The school can even propose to pay a part of the costs of smoking cessation interventions, which will demonstrate the school's commitment to helping employees who use tobacco. Providing smoking cessation programmes is expensive and requires a commitment of resources that many schools do not have. Or, a school can collaborate with health services to provide smoking cessation and/or self-help cessation materials to employees. This alternative takes advantage of existing resources and does not require a continuing effort by the employer, though it does require a start-up effort by the school.

Yet another alternative is to provide referral

information about community smoking cessation programmes or self-help cessation materials for employees. This option also takes advantage of using existing resources and will be less expensive than the first two options. It will also be easier to implement because it requires less school effort. However, this option will have less effect on tobacco use and health care costs.

Abstaining from tobacco use does not in itself guarantee good health. Excluding tobacco is an important part of a healthy lifestyle that also includes physical exercise. Physical exercise, recreation and sport help individuals acquire and maintain physical fitness and serve as a healthy means of self-expression and social development. Physical exercise, instead of tobacco use, offers alternatives for dealing with stress and being accepted by peers.

Physical exercise, recreation and sport can also show the negative consequences of tobacco use on the body because tobacco can impede physical and aerobic performance. It is also a way to show improvement in physical condition after quitting tobacco use. Recreational activities can restore strength and spirits during and after school and work. Ball games, dances or trips can support good health and offer opportunities for reducing stress and spending time with peers or colleagues.

An individual's psychological well-being, including self-esteem and self-confidence, is critical to tobacco use prevention. School counselling programmes and social support provide guidance for students, school personnel and families in dealing with difficulties, adjustments, growth and development. Education about life skills teaches decision-making skills, stress management and refusal skills.

Role of Teachers and Staffs

Teachers and other school staff are intermediaries who can address tobacco use prevention with young people in powerful ways. They are in daily contact with students and provide means and facilities to structure fragmented knowledge in a systematic way. Teachers provide a structured way of learning that helps students acquire necessary knowledge, attitudes and skills to adopt a healthy lifestyle.

Tobacco use interventions can only be effective if teachers are actively involved in developing and implementing such interventions. In all communities, the training of teachers should be of highest priority because teachers provide the information to students and serve as role models for their students. In addition, teachers traditionally play an influential role in their communities.

Their own behaviours and actions can promote positive attitudes outside the classroom. Thus, it is important to train teachers and other school personnel to implement tobacco use interventions, and, if necessary, offer them a tobacco use cessation programme so they can set a healthy example as non-tobacco users.

Adequate curriculum implementation and overall programme effectiveness are enhanced when teachers are trained to deliver the programme as planned. Teachers need to be trained to recognize the importance of carefully and completely implementing the selected programme, and become familiar with its underlying theory and conceptual framework. Training for teachers and other school personnel should involve:

— *a rationale for implementing tobacco use prevention and reduction interventions in schools*

— *allocation of authority, personnel, time and resources to a staff member who will be responsible for initiating, managing and coordinating training*

— *regularly scheduled follow-up sessions that provide updates about the status of tobacco use and progress in reducing and preventing the initiation of tobacco use*

— *the development of a core training group who will enable all relevant teachers and school personnel to receive training in a timely manner*

— *an evaluation to determine how confident teachers and other school personnel feel about preventing and reducing tobacco use*

Because health education involves influencing attitudes, values and skills, as well as knowledge to promote healthy behaviours and conditions, teachers must be trained to use a wide variety of teaching methods. Some teachers rely on one or two educational methods, such as lectures and worksheets. Although these methods may reach a large number of people and convey vast amounts of information that might otherwise not be disseminated, lectures are not very effective in helping to build prevention skills.

Teacher training should focus on methods that engage students and parents in the educational process, such as discussion, debates, role playing and community education projects. All these training elements can help ensure the effectiveness and relevance of tobacco use interventions.

Sun Protection in Health Promoting Schools

Ultra Violet (UV) radiation is one component of the many different types of radiation emitted by the sun (sometimes described as the solar spectrum); it is also produced by artificial sources, such as tanning lamps and solariums. Unlike visible light, which can be detected by our eyes and the infrared radiation that gives the sun its heat, UV radiation can neither be seen nor felt.

The intensity of solar UV radiation is influenced by the following:

— *Sun height: The higher the sun in the sky, the higher the UV level. Thus, UV levels vary with time of day and time of year, with maximum levels generally occurring when the sun is directly overhead (solar noon), which is around midday in the summer (although this depends on location and whether daylight savings time is used).*

— *Latitude: The closer to the equator, the higher the UV levels.*

— *Cloud cover: Heavy clouds can significantly reduce UV levels, whilst scattered clouds result in levels rising and falling as clouds pass in front of the sun. Even with cloud cover, UV levels can be high due to the scattering of UV radiation by particles of moisture and other materials in the atmosphere.*

— *Ozone:* Ozone absorbs some of the UV radiation that would otherwise reach the earth's surface. Ozone levels vary throughout the year and even across the day.

— *Altitude:* At higher altitudes, a thinner atmosphere filters less UV radiation. Thus, with every 1,000 meters altitude, UV levels can increase by approximately 8 percent.

— *Environment:* UV is reflected or scattered to varying extents by different surfaces. For example, snow can reflect as much as 80 percent of UV radiation; dry beach sand, about 15 percent. UV radiation that has been scattered or reflected is sometimes referred to as indirect UV.

Health effects of UV exposure

The sun is the vital source of energy for all life on this planet. It would be impossible to survive without the sun. Exposure to sunlight enables the body to produce vitamin D, which plays a crucial role in skeletal development, immune function, and blood cell formation. However, 10 to 15 minutes daily exposure of face, forearms, and hands to normal Northern European summer sun is sufficient to maintain vitamin D levels.

Closer to the equator, where UV levels are higher, even shorter periods of exposure suffice. Hence, for most people, vitamin D deficiency is unlikely. Possible exceptions are those who have very limited sun exposure (e.g., the housebound elderly), or those with heavily pigmented skin who live in areas where UV levels are relatively low. The UV spectrum can be *divided into three different categories: UVA, UVB, and UVC. UVC does not reach the earth's surface. Both UVA and UVB radiation are responsible for harmful effects on the skin, eyes, and immune system.*

In the short term, excessive exposure to UV radiation causes sunburn-reddening (erythema), pain, and, in severe cases, blistering of the skin. Over time, UV exposure, whether or not it is associated with sunburn, accelerates skin ageing and causes changes in body cells, which may lead to skin cancer. There are three different forms of skin cancer, each named for the type of skin cell in which they originate:

— *Basal cell carcinoma: the most common and least dangerous skin cancer*

— *Squamous cell carcinoma: the type that may spread to other parts of the body if not treated*

— *Melanoma: the least common but most dangerous form of skin cancer, which, if not treated quickly, releases cancer cells that spread to other parts of the body (i.e., metastasise), possibly resulting in death Basal and squamous cell carcinomas are often referred to collectively as common or non-melanocytic skin cancers (NMSCs).*

UV radiation also causes changes at the cellular and molecular level that result in the suppression of immune function, thereby compromising the body's ability to resist disease. Exposure of the eyes to UV radiation over long periods contributes to the development of cataracts (i.e., cloudiness of the lens that can ultimately result in blindness) and pterygium (i.e., an overgrowth of the conjunctiva onto the cornea).

The incidence of skin cancer has increased since the early 1970s, by as much as 4 percent per year in the United States; skin cancer represents one in every three cancers diagnosed globally. This increase has been attributed to changes in behaviour, such as increased participation in outdoor activities and more frequent sunbathing. Changes in travel patterns may also contribute to increases in sun exposure and therefore skin cancer incidence.

High levels of the skin pigment melanin appear to reduce the risk of common skin cancers for people with darker skin; however, in the case of severe sun exposure, melanin appears to be less effective in protecting against melanoma. Moreover, when skin cancer occurs in people with darker skin, it is likely to be detected later, when the cancer is more advanced and therefore more dangerous. Excessive exposure to UV radiation is an issue of global concern, as eye damage and immune suppression affect all skin types equally.

Some 12 to 15 million people are blind from cataracts, and, according to WHO estimates, up to 20 percent of these may be caused or enhanced by sun exposure, especially in countries located close to the equator, such as India and Pakistan. The possibilities of increased risk of infection and reduced efficacy of immunization as a result of UV exposure have serious global implications. Again, the most vulnerable population are children living in countries located close to the equator.

Development and implementation of sun protection strategies should also have beneficial effects for the immune competence of those at added risk of infection as a result of UV exposure. The key element of sun protection is minimizing the amount of time spent in the sun, particularly during the period when UV radiation is at its most intense, generally the four hour period around solar noon. When possible, indoor activities should be planned for this period.

Outdoor activities should always be organized to make the maximum possible use of shade. When outdoors, as much of the skin should be protected as possible with loose fitting, tightly woven clothing. Garments with at least elbow length sleeves and collars, and longer skirts or trousers are most effective. Headwear should shade the face, the back of the neck, and the ears, such as a hat with a brim of about 8-10 cm or a legionnaire style cap with flaps on the back and sides.

Sunscreen should be used for areas that cannot be adequately covered with clothing, including the face, which is only partially protected by a hat. Even in the shade, indirect UV levels can be sufficiently high to be harmful, so sunscreen should be worn at all times when outdoors. To provide protection against UVA and UVB, a broad spectrum sunscreen with a sun protection factor (SPF) of at least 15 is recommended. Even when applied correctly, no sunscreen is able to block UV radiation completely, so it should never be used as the first or only method of sun protection. It also should not be used to extend the amount of time spent in the sun, or in place of clothing.

There is strong evidence that exposure to UV radiation during childhood and adolescence is a risk factor for developing skin cancer later in life. It is also estimated that the majority of a person's lifetime UV exposure occurs during childhood. Protecting young people's skin and eyes should reduce future incidence of skin cancer and eye problems. Children are also the group most susceptible to the effects of reduced immune competence because of their greater vulnerability to infections. The development of good habits during childhood can also contribute to more appropriate sun behaviour later in life, and thus to a further overall reduction in lifetime UV exposure.

Importance of Sun protection during Childhood

UV exposure during the school years contributes significantly to total lifetime exposure During the first 18 years of life, when much of one's lifetime UV exposure is received, a significant proportion of time is spent at school or participating in school based activities, such as camps or school sports. Students attend school for most of the year, and school hours generally incorporate peak UV periods.

Some school events, such as sporting carnivals, can require students, staff, and spectators to be outdoors for the entire school day. Outdoor activities and break times, particularly lunch, frequently occur at times when UV levels are at their maximum. Thus, the school environment and the manner in which a school operates can have a significant impact on children's UV exposure at the period in their lives when they are most vulnerable to its effects.

Structural and organizational strategies that provide sun protection for students and staff while they are at school are simple to adopt and can also be used to compensate to some extent for the reluctance of adolescents to adopt personal sun protection measures. For example, providing attractive shaded areas that are likely to be used by adolescents for passive recreation during breaks can reduce the need for use of protective clothing at these times.

Implementation of such strategies also provides a practical demonstration of how such measures can be adopted beyond the school environment. For example, ensuring that sun protection strategies are an integral component of all outdoor activities, including school breaks and sports lessons, illustrates to students and parents how sun protection can be incorporated into other family and community activities.

Schools are vitally important settings through which to promote education about UV radiation and providing sun protection It is important to target children's attitudes and behaviour at a young age, particularly in primary school, when children tend to be most receptive to the need for sun protection-during adolescence, influences of peers and fashion are more likely to take precedence.

School programmes can not only help to reduce UV exposure at school, but also to facilitate the development of habits and attitudes that can have an impact on sun exposure at other times. Because children of school age have more leisure time, much of which tends to be spent outdoors, good habits carried over from the school setting can further contribute to reductions in total UV exposure.

Role modeling of appropriate sun behaviour by staff is a vital element in educating students and parents as well as protecting staff from excessive UV exposure, but the school can also become a role model for families and other community organizations, such as sporting clubs or kindergartens. Having to plan for sun protection at school can make it easier for parents and students to plan for sun protection during activities that occur outside the school environment.

Personal sun protection equipment is simple and readily portable-a hat, a shirt, and sunscreen can be carried from one venue to another in a small bag. Curriculum programmes focusing on or incorporating sun protection education can be used to develop communication and life skills. These are ideally part of a comprehensive approach that aims to develop positive attitudes toward preventive measures and to promote responsible decision making, all of which are essential for general health and well-being.

Because reducing UV exposure is a more specific objective than, for example, "healthy eating", and personal sun protection strategies are quite easy to implement, sun protection education can be used as a starting point prior to tackling some of the broader, more complex issues (such as nutrition).

Sensible sun exposure behaviour contributes to decreasing the risks of some of today's leading health problems UV exposure causes sunburn, accelerates skin ageing, and is the major risk factor for the development of skin cancer. It also contributes to eye damage and suppresses immune function. Hence, reducing exposure to UV radiation is an issue of global concern. It has been estimated that more than 2 million non-melanoma skin cancers and 200,000 malignant melanomas occur globally each year-one in every three cancers diagnosed is skin cancer.

Given levels of ozone depletion and current trends, it is predicted that this will increase by as much as 300,000 non-melanoma skin cancers and 4,500 melanomas each year. However, appropriate sun exposure behaviour could prevent as many as four out of five cases of skin cancer. High levels of skin cancer in Australia, Europe, and the United States have resulted in campaigns designed specifically to reduce UV exposure.

In Australia, where skin cancer is the most common form of cancer, there is evidence that public health campaigns conducted over the past 20 years to reduce sun exposure may be having a beneficial effect on skin cancer rates. It has also been estimated that up to 20 percent of the 12 to 15 million cases of blindness due to cataracts can be at least partially attributed to UV exposure, particularly in countries located near the equator.

Consequently, 3 million people's sight may be saved each year through the use of appropriate eye protection. Moreover, a 10 percent decrease in total ozone levels is predicted to result in between 1.6 and 1.75 million additional cases of cataracts per year worldwide. The growing evidence that UV exposure can also result in reduced effectiveness of the immune system has serious implications for the efficacy of immunization programmes and the spread of infection, particularly for many Asian, African, and South American countries.

Preventive health habits developed at a young age are likely to continue into adulthood Sun protection strategies are relatively easy to adopt and incorporate into a daily routine, to the extent that they become habits. If these behaviours are regularly reinforced and role modeled, they are more likely to continue into adulthood, particularly as children's capacity to understand the reasons for such habits increases.

Knowing how to prevent a recurrence of sunburn can provide children with a sense of control over their own health and well-being. Most children are capable of putting on hats as they go outside and, with guidance and practice, can learn to correctly apply sunscreen. These simple strategies can quickly become part of the daily routine. Another helpful factor is that, unlike other preventive measures, where the effects may not become evident for several years, the symptoms of sunburn are more immediate, thus enabling children to relate the behaviour (lack of sun protection) to the outcome (sunburn).

School children are especially susceptible to fashion trends suggesting that a suntan is healthy. The influence of peer pressure and fashion becomes more powerful during adolescence, and good habits tend to be replaced by sun seeking behaviours. This is often based on the belief that a tan is healthy and attractive; it is also at least partially due to the fact that, with the possible exception of sunglasses, sun protective clothing is seldom considered fashionable by young people.

Even when adolescents are aware of the long term implications, they tend to be reluctant to protect themselves, just as they are more likely to indulge in other forms of risk taking behaviour, such as tobacco use or unprotected sex. It is important to address these issues through programmes that develop life skills, promote healthy decision making, and give young people the self-esteem to address these pressures. Such programmes may also help to change the group norms that are a factor in the rejection of personal sun protection.

Surveys of Australian secondary school students suggest that the proportion seeking a dark tan had decreased, and those seeking a light tan increased between 1990 and 1996. This suggests that awareness of the need for sun protection can positively influence attitudes and behaviour, even in this age group. Although the majority of young people still indicate that they do seek a tan, it is a step in the right direction.

Reducing sun exposure enables healthy adulthood and ageing. In the short term, excessive exposure to UV radiation causes sunburn. The symptoms, although painful, seldom last more than a few days, except in severe cases. However, childhood UV exposure is a major factor in the development of skin cancer later in life. Children must therefore be a key target group for prevention programmes.

Non-melanoma skin cancers tend to develop around age 40, and melanoma can affect people in their late teens and early 20s. In Australia, melanoma is the most common cancer in the 15-44 years age group. Since those who have been diagnosed with skin cancer are considered to be at greater risk of developing it again, the disease can potentially affect a person's health for a significant proportion of his or her lifetime.

Sun exposure also causes other skin damage, including wrinkling, pigmentation changes, and other non-malignant lesions. These can become apparent from a relatively early age. Reducing childhood exposure should reduce the incidence of such problems during adulthood and, if good habits are maintained for much of the lifetime, should improve the health of older individuals.

Similarly, use of eye protection is likely to delay the onset of cataracts and to reduce the incidence of blindness from cataracts. This has obvious implications for the health and well-being of adults, not the least of which is the preservation of their independence, something that is extremely important to older people.

Investing in sun protection interventions decreases costs in the health system and strengthens the economy. In Australia, skin cancer is the most costly of all cancers to the Australian health system. The direct costs of treatment have been estimated at US$5.70 per head per annum, while the cost of current prevention campaigns has been calculated at US$0.08 per head per annum. Assuming that a 20 year prevention campaign costing US$0.17 per head per annum reduced UV radiation exposure by 20 percent, and that melanoma rates began to fall after a 5 year lag, and that non-melanocytic skin cancers and solar keratoses fell after a 15 year lag, the predicted annual savings would be US$0.17 per person. In other words, every dollar spent would save a dollar in health care costs.

India has a particularly high incidence of cataracts, a significant percentage of which are likely to be related to UV exposure, and in 1994 was granted US$118 million by the World Bank to reduce its backlog in cataract surgery. Considerable savings are therefore possible if the development of cataracts can be prevented or delayed. With ongoing ozone depletion, UV levels on earth are likely to rise and people will experience more harmful UV exposure It has been predicted that depletion of the ozone layer, due to the *release of substances such as chlorofluorocarbons (CFCs), will result in an increase in the amounts of UV radiation reaching the earth's surface.*

There are also seasonal holes in the ozone layer over the Antarctic and the Arctic, which contribute to higher UV levels at particular times of the year. While there is considerable uncertainty about the implications for human health, an increase in UV related problems such as skin and eye damage is a potential consequence, particularly in the Northern Hemisphere, where the "hole" is more likely to extend over heavily populated areas.

The Montreal Protocol, an agreement limiting the use of chemicals that destroy the ozone, should result in a reduction in the rate at which this damage occurs, provided that there is full compliance. However, even if compliance is complete, it is expected that the ozone layer will not recover until at least the middle of the 21st century. During 2000, the ozone hole over the Antarctic extended over such populated areas as Chile, where residents were warned that they could get sunburned in less than seven minutes due to increased UV levels.

Furthermore, it is now believed that ozone damage may be exacerbated by the greenhouse effect, despite reductions in levels of ozone depleting chemicals in the atmosphere. Given the uncertainties relating to the possible health consequences of ozone depletion, it is clear that taking action to reduce UV exposure is essential. The only way to protect people against the possible risks associated with ozone damage is to encourage them to protect themselves.

In view of the sensitivity of children's skin, it is even more critical that action is taken to reduce childhood exposure to UV. We can improve health and well-being through sun protection in schools. There is evidence that school based interventions are effective in improving levels of sun protection for children in younger grade levels. In Australia, this has resulted in the development of the National SunSmart Schools Programme, which seeks to provide a consistent, high standard approach to sun protection across all primary schools.

The key elements of effective sun protection interventions in schools are considered to be the following:

— *Development of a comprehensive sun protection policy that clearly documents strategies:*

— *Involving parents and students in the policy development process is important to secure their support and improve their understanding of the strategies.*

Effective school sun protection involves a holistic approach that employs strategies that address behaviour, the curriculum, and the environment. The Health-Promoting Schools model provides an ideal framework within which to implement a comprehensive approach to sun protection. Schools can provide interventions to improve sun protection in ways that are highly cost effective Interventions to improve sun protection are relatively simple to implement and, in most cases, inexpensive.

Changes to school uniforms or dress codes can be phased in over a period of time and incorporate clothing (including sunglasses) that can be worn outside the school environment. Sunscreen can be purchased in bulk by schools to reduce the cost to students, but, as awareness and understanding increases, this may be an item that parents are willing to purchase for their children anyway, for use not just at school but also at other times.

While shade development is often costly, it can be incorporated in a broader environmental programme. For example, tree planting can be promoted not just as a means of improving shade, but also of enhancing air and soil quality. Shade, whether provided by trees or structures, also has other obvious benefits in improving the overall school environment.

Shade development can also be a process that fosters more active parental participation through, for example, fundraising activities. Active involvement of children in the process can provide them with practical experience in setting and working toward shared goals, and perhaps even become the foundation for participation in similar activities at the community level. Such participation can enhance students' sense of ownership of the outcome and help to develop their confidence and communication skills. Changes to scheduling of outdoor activities can be achieved relatively cheaply or at no cost.

For example, extending the morning break and having it at a time when UV levels are lower, and shortening the lunch break, which usually occurs at the peak UV time, is cost neutral. There can even be benefits; for example, beginning sporting carnivals in the late afternoon may increase parental participation. Simple, low cost activities can be used to educate children and their families about UV radiation and sun protection.

In fact, children can gradually take on the task of educating other members of their family and the wider community. This can give them pride in their knowledge, as well as a sense of control over their own health and that of others close to them. Apart from reducing sun exposure of students while they are at school, these interventions serve to educate staff and parents and can readily be applied to situations beyond the school environment. For example, hats and shirts with collars can be incorporated into uniforms for community sporting clubs, and a tree planting programme could be introduced for a local sports ground.

Sun protection education for girls has a positive impact on the health of families Improving the health and education of girls is likely to improve that of their children, because girls or women generally have most of the responsibility for supervision, education, and care of other members of their households. Teaching girls why and how to minimize UV exposure not only reduces their own risk of harmful effects on the skin, eye, and immune system, but also provides them with simple strategies to protect other members of their families and, in particular, their own children.

Almost equally important is the enhancement of their own self-esteem and confidence as a result of their greater ability to control factors affecting their health and that of others. Sun protection interventions in schools benefit the entire community Schools are often the hub of their communities-a venue for local events and a meeting point for parents. Elements of sun protection, such as hat wearing and shade development are highly visible, and, as such, implementation of these strategies can demonstrate good practice to the broader community.

The school can act as a model for other community organizations and groups; activities in the area of sun protection may be an entry point for schools to adopt a more pro active role in the community with respect to other health issues. As teachers are often active members of their communities-for example, as users of child care or preschools, or as members of sporting clubs-they are able to take their knowledge and experiences and apply them in the broader community setting.

Schools are also one means of introducing new health information and partnerships between the school and local organizations, groups, and businesses, which can benefit all members of the community. For example, a local business may offer discounts on sunscreen and hats in return for promotion through school newsletters and bulletins; community health workers may conduct sun protection education programmes in schools.

As a health issue with a very specific risk factor, sun protection is ideal as an entry point to becoming a Health-Promoting School. If this has already been achieved, sun protection interventions are readily incorporated within the Health-Promoting School Framework. The first step in developing interventions to minimize UV exposure is to decide that this is a health and educational priority. It is then necessary to plan the interventions by determining which strategies will have the most significant impact on health and education, and how these strategies can be integrated with other health promotion activities to best effect.

Health-Promoting Schools involve members of the school and community in planning programmes that respond to their needs and can be maintained with available resources and commitments. Establishing a school health team and a community advisory committee are important steps in the planning process. The school health team is responsible for the coordination and monitoring of health promotion policies and activities.

It is essential that parents, students, and staff, including management, are involved in the planning process from the outset. If such a team does not exist, the introduction of sun protection interventions can be the stimulus for its formation and provide a model on which other health interventions may be based. Student involvement is essential in order to develop strategies that are relevant to student needs and concerns and will enlist their support.

Effective sun protection relies to a significant extent on student cooperation, which is most likely to be achieved if students actively participate in the decision making process and feel a sense of ownership. Parental input is also critical to ensure that strategies are feasible; i.e., parents must be willing and able to support the purchase of hats, sunglasses, and sunscreen and possibly to assist in shade development.

As school staff are primarily responsible for implementation, their input is essential in order to ensure that strategies are practical within the context of the school environment, organization, and available resources. The school health team should include a balance of young people and adults with an interest in and commitment to the well-being of the school community, for example, students, teachers, administrators, and parents.

This team must be given the time, resources, and authority to enable it to lead and oversee health promotion activities in the school. A sun protection working group that is a sub committee of this team would have responsibility for the planning and implementation of sun protection interventions.

Community advisory committee is also important to work with groups or individuals outside the school who have an interest in health promotion and may influence student knowledge, attitudes, and behaviour in relation to UV exposure and sun protection. If such a committee does not already exist, development of a sun protection intervention can be an opportunity to establish one. Potential partners might include local government representatives, businesses, community youth agencies, nongovernmental organizations, health service providers, and sporting groups.

The committee should include people with a range of skills, interests, and resources who can assist the school health team in the implementation of sun protection interventions. The team should also represent the community's geographical, economic, social, ethnic, and religious composition. To facilitate the efforts of the school health team, there are a number of things the community advisory committee can do:

— *Help determine local needs and resources*

— *Disseminate information about UV exposure and the need for sun protection*

— *Build support across the community*

— *Encourage community involvement*

— *Help obtain resources and funding for sun protection interventions*

— *Reinforce learning experiences provided in the school*

The community advisory committee and the school health team should work together in planning health promotion efforts and in coordinating the various components of a Health-Promoting School, such as health education, health services, and community and family involvement, in order to maximize health outcomes.

To be effective, sun protection interventions require commitment and action from a wide range of individuals and groups. It is also important to obtain the support of relevant government departments, health and education authorities, community and business leaders, educators, parents, students, and the community.

Sun protection interventions in schools are greatly facilitated by support at various levels of government and from the ministries of health and education. Efforts to achieve effective sun protection interventions in the context of a Health-Promoting School also rely on community understanding and support. It is essential that parents and community members participate in the design, content, delivery, and evaluation of interventions.

This should occur from the outset to ensure that families and the community have the opportunity to raise any concerns and to participate in the planning process. Such involvement is also important to create a sense of community ownership and to enable resources, facilities, and expertise to be shared effectively. It can be achieved through community group meetings, formal presentations, individual meetings with relevant groups and individuals use of school publications, and even local media.

School Policies

School policies provide the framework for the implementation of sun protection interventions. Policies should be simple statements of the rationale, objectives, and guidelines for implementation relating to the school environment, behaviour, and curriculum. They may also incorporate statements about the policy evaluation process. They should take into account specific factors that may influence implementation, such as local climatic conditions, and times of day and/or year at which UV levels are sufficiently high to constitute a risk.

Policy development requires input from teachers and administrators, parents and students, and all other relevant members of the school community. It should take into consideration other relevant health concerns and health promotion activities, as well as the needs, priorities, and cultural practices of groups represented in the school community. Collaboration between the school and the community and with relevant health and government authorities is strongly recommended.

The following rules or guidelines could be included in a sun protection policy:

— *Teachers, parents, students and all other relevant*

school personnel will be represented in the planning, development and review process.

- *The community advisory committee will meet periodically to maintain coordination between the school and community.*
- *Teachers will receive ongoing training in relation to appropriate sun protection strategies.*
- *The school is committed to ensuring that sufficient shade is available within its grounds.*
- *The school encourages the use of shade as a means of reducing UV exposure during outdoor activities.*
- *Outdoor activities will be minimized during periods when UV radiation is at its most intense.*
- *Students, teachers, other staff, and parents will wear sun protective clothing whilst involved in outdoor activities organized by/for the school.*
- *The need for sun protection for participants and spectators will be reflected in the planning for all outdoor events conducted by or at the school, e.g., by choosing venues that have adequate shade.*
- *Sun protection education will be included sequentially as part of a comprehensive school health programme.*
- *The school will encourage the use of maximum protection sunscreen as a method of sun protection, to be used properly and in conjunction with other methods, especially for areas of skin that cannot adequately be protected by clothing and hats, including the face.*
- *Parents will be educated about the need for a*

combination of sun protection methods for themselves and their families during outdoor activities.

Goals and objectives of sun protection

Goals and objectives are essential to guide and clarify what the sun protection interventions are intended to achieve and how the interventions are to be evaluated. Goals and objectives should be developed by the school health team in collaboration with the community advisory committee, on the basis of the situation analysis.

The goals should describe in broad terms what the programme will achieve. The goals of sun protection interventions in a Health-Promoting School should include, but not be limited to, these three:

- *To provide a school environment that reduces the UV exposure of students, and other members of the school, the students' families, and the community*
- *To develop knowledge of and attitudes toward sun protection that will result in adoption of sun protection behaviours by students and other members of the school, the students' families, and the community*
- *To develop the skills, behaviours, and confidence that will be the basis of lifelong sun protection habits*

The goals are then broken down into specific outcome and process objectives so that everyone clearly understands what needs to be done, when, and why. Objectives are the steps for reaching an overall goal;

they describe outcomes in measurable terms that will help determine how successfully the goal is being reached.

A Health-Promoting School strives to use the school's full organizational capacity to improve the health of students, school personnel, families, and community members. Such a school offers many opportunities to promote sun protection as an essential element for the attainment of health. Sun protection interventions can serve as an entry point for the development or enhancement of policies, planning groups, and various components, which serve as a framework for a Health-Promoting School. These components include, but are not limited to:

- *skills based health education*
- *a healthy school environment*
- *school safety*
- *school health services*
- *physical exercise, recreation, and sports*
- *community and family involvement and outreach*
- *counseling and social support health*
- *promotion for school staff*

The effectiveness of the interventions integrated into each of the above components is influenced by the extent to which they are supported by a variety of people, policies and trained staff. Their effectiveness is also influenced by the extent to which interventions in each of these components combine with other health promotion efforts to complement and reinforce one another.

Not all schools will have the resources to integrate sun protection interventions into all of the components at one time. Therefore, each school has to establish its own priorities, in collaboration with all parties concerned, and decide the extent to which the components should be addressed. A Health-Promoting School enables students, parents, teachers, and community members to work together to make such decisions. It is more important to start with small changes that are possible than to wait until resources become available to address all components simultaneously.

School health education should help individuals avoid health risks and create an environment that is conducive to health for all. Thus, behaviours and conditions that are to be influenced must be clearly defined. Common behaviours that should be addressed to prevent or reduce the risk of UV related health problems include the following:

— *Unprotected exposure during breaks*

— *Unprotected exposure when travelling to and from school*

— *Unprotected exposure during organized outdoor activities*

— *Outdoor activities conducted during peak UV periods*

— *Inappropriate use of sunscreens*

Close collaboration between education and health officials, the School Health Team, the Community Advisory Committee, and other school and community members is necessary to identify the particular behaviours and conditions relevant to health in each community. In a Health-Promoting School, sun protection education is designed to help students acquire the knowledge, attitudes, beliefs, and skills they need to make informed decisions, practice healthy behaviours and create conditions conducive to health.

In a Health-Promoting School, skills based health education about sun protection addresses the nature of UV radiation and its beneficial and harmful effects on health and well-being. It also provides strategies to minimize of UV exposure in the context of a healthy lifestyle, which necessarily includes outdoor activities.

It should provide opportunities for students to acquire the knowledge they need to make informed decisions about their exposure to UV radiation from the sun and other sources. It should also enable them to critically evaluate and question images that present a suntan as a sign of good health and attractiveness.

Skills based health education should occur sequentially from primary through secondary levels, addressing the physical, mental, emotional, and social dimensions of health. It can be taught as a specific subject, as part of several subjects, or ideally a combination of both. Sun protection education should be part of the school health curriculum and should be integrated into a range of subject areas.

The most obvious of these is science, where, for example, the nature of UV radiation can be explored; students can investigate the structure and function of the skin, the eye, and the immune system, and the effects of UV radiation on each. However, it can also be part of a number of other subject areas.

Sun protection education should also be incorporated into the school's extracurricular activities, particularly outdoor events, and integrated into other school health components, such as physical activity and staff health. Appropriate scheduling of sun protection education, taking into consideration factors such as latitude, climate, lifestyle and cultural factors, enhances its relevance for students.

Children's understanding of sun protection messages is enhanced and reinforced by experience of warm, sunny weather and the practice of taking care in the sun. Often, spring will be the best time of year to incorporate sun protection education, however it may also be relevant prior to the skiing season or a holiday period. Sun protection education should be combined with efforts addressing other health issues, as appropriate.

For example, a primary school programme on safety could include such topics as road safety, hygiene, and safe behaviour in the sun. A secondary school programme on healthy decision making could incorporate critical discussion of images of good health and attractiveness relating to body shape, tanning, and tobacco use. A variety of issues can be addressed simultaneously, with specific issues explored in greater depth to make a particular point. Alternatively, by coordinating or linking the presentation of related topics in different classes, the issues can be linked, and learning experiences can reinforce and complement one another.

Linking of sun protection issues with other relevant topics can also be enhanced by co-teaching, sharing teaching resources, referring students to related lessons, and involving students from different classes in different activities. Curriculum resources for sun protection education may be available through governmental and nongovernmental agencies and organizations, universities, or teacher's unions.

In selecting essential knowledge for students in relation to UV radiation and sun protection, information that will enable students to make and act on sensible decisions regarding sun protection, rather than technical information in relation to the nature of UV radiation or sun protection methods, should be emphasized. For example, students being able to apply sunscreen effectively is more important than their ability to explain how the SPF for sunscreen is determined.

There should be opportunities to develop skills and knowledge that can be applied at school, at home, and in the community. For example, students can actively participate in the design of school uniforms or the development of a sun safe school dress code, and they can develop a plan to reduce UV exposure for participants in a favourite leisure activity.

Training is an essential prerequisite for school personnel involved in the development, implementation, and delivery of school health education programmes. Ideally, training should be ongoing and incorporate time for personnel to receive accurate information, discuss issues, share ideas and resources, and evaluate programmes. Opportunities should be available for teachers to develop their own skills in the kinds of teaching strategies necessary to influence attitudes and beliefs and develop skills, rather than simply focusing on knowledge.

Teachers need to be both competent and confident

in using such strategies as discussions, debates, role plays, practical activities, and community education projects. Such strategies are sometimes avoided by teachers because they can be more time consuming and difficult to manage than conventional methods; they must also be well planned and executed if they are to achieve their objectives. Therefore, it is important that teachers are given the opportunity to develop and practice these necessary skills.

In a Health-Promoting School, health education may be integrated across several curriculum areas, and thus teachers in all curriculum areas should be encouraged to incorporate health issues into their programmes. Furthermore, all personnel have a responsibility to act as role models for students by demonstrating appropriate sun protection behaviours; in doing so, they will be seen by students as supportive of sun protection interventions and therefore understand the rationale underlying the strategies the school implements.

Finally, school personnel should understand why sun protection is necessary and how to protect themselves for their own health and well-being. Their duties often require them to participate in activities that increase their exposure to UV radiation, and it is important that they understand both the risks and how to minimize them. Additional components relating to, for example, the importance of early detection of skin cancer should also be incorporated, as appropriate.

In Northern latitude countries, the potential for excessive sun exposure poses a health risk for only a relatively short period of each year. As a consequence, health risks of UV radiation exposure are often not perceived as important or relevant in the school context. With an already packed curriculum many teachers may decide to concentrate their limited time and resources on key curricular activities.

Participation and empowerment are key principles of a Health-Promoting School. Students should be involved in planning school health programmes, carrying out the activities, and evaluating them in a structured way. There are several ways in which students can be actively engaged and empowered:

— *Involving them in policy development: Ensuring that students participate in the decision making process-for example, through student councils or representative bodies-is essential to gain their support.*

— *Involving them in the development and evaluation of implementation strategies:*

Strategies developed by students are more likely to receive student support. For example, students can redesign components of the school uniform to increase the level of sun protection provided, or design and build a new shade structure for the school grounds-thus achieving a sense of ownership in the outcomes. Students may offer creative solutions or strategies that are more likely to be accepted by other students because they understand what is relevant and important to young people.

Students can also act as role models through more specific educational activities, for example, by developing and implementing education programmes for other students. However, peer educators must be properly trained to ensure that they have not just the knowledge but also the skills necessary to support other students.

Participating in community education and other community projects: Important community links can be developed through student participation in programmes involving the wider community. This might include, for example, conducting information sessions for families, organizing a tree planting programme for a local recreational facility, or helping to develop a sun protection policy for a sports club.

For sustainable improvements in levels of sun protection, the Health-Promoting School must create an environment that supports interventions through changes, not just to the physical environment, but also through policies and practices. The physical environment is made up of the school buildings, classrooms, and school grounds, including areas used for passive and active recreation. The condition of the physical environment can have a significant impact on the UV exposure levels of members of the school community.

Three key aspects of the physical environment should be addressed:

Shade: It is essential that students and staff have access to adequate shaded areas. In particular, shade must be available at peak UV periods, that is, during the middle of the day, for outdoor activities and also, if appropriate, for breaks. This is especially important if students are expected to eat lunch outside-it should be possible for all students to eat their lunch in the shade, or alternatives should be offered, for example, allowing students to eat in classrooms before going outside. Shaded areas should also be sufficiently attractive so that students will be willing to use them, for example, by providing seating and keeping the area clean. Where possible, shade should be incorporated into building design, for example, by using verandas and covered walkways. Tree planting is a cheaper, more long term solution than shade structures, and is a means of significantly improving the atmosphere of the school; however, temporary measures may be needed until new trees are able to provide adequate protection.

Clothing: Clothing that provides effective sun protection should be available to students, staff, and parents and its use encouraged or required. Recommended items include broad brimmed or legionnaire hats; shirts with collars and longer sleeves; longer style shorts, skirts, or trousers; and wrap around sunglasses with UV protective lenses. Clothing used for sporting activities is particularly important, as students are often outdoors for extended periods during such activities.

Scheduling of outdoor activities: Where possible, outdoor activities should be scheduled to avoid peak UV periods and to make the best possible use of shaded areas or indoor facilities. This also includes events that involve students spending extended periods of time outdoors, such as sporting carnivals. Beginning such events later in the day or conducting them over successive mornings can help to avoid excessive UV exposure. Midday breaks can be shortened and morning or late afternoon breaks extended to minimize the amount of time spent outdoors during peak UV periods.

The psychosocial environment relates to the social and mental conditions that affect education and health. The ambience of a Health-Promoting School is one that respects the individual and fosters confidence in healthy lifestyles. The following aspects of a healthy psychosocial environment should be integrated into a Health-Promoting School:

Teacher role models: Teachers play an important role as adult role models and mentors. Teachers can encourage students to protect themselves from the sun by wearing protective clothing and sunscreen and seeking shade. This applies particularly to physical education/sports teachers who are often key role models for popular students and student leaders. If student leaders are positively influenced, they can in turn influence others.

Peer reinforcement: Students can provide positive reinforcement to their peers by showing that sun seeking behaviour is not a requirement for peer acceptance. Schools therefore need to provide time and opportunities to enable students to socialize in environments where UV exposure is avoided or minimized.

School health services help foster health and well-being as well as prevent, reduce, monitor, and treat important health problems or conditions. In Health-Promoting Schools, health services and are provided to students, school personnel, families, and community members, and are coordinated with other sun protection services and activities in the school and community.

One role of a school health service may be the provision of sunscreen, which should be available for all school activities. In deciding how to make sunscreen available, schools should consider five things:

Access: Schools can request that sunscreen be

applied prior to students coming to school, and make provisions for reapplication during the day. Schools may also request parents to supply sunscreen; however, a school supply should always be available.

Choice of sunscreen: Sunscreen should have an SPF of at least 15, protect against both UVA and UVB, and preferably be water resistant.

Skin reactions: Due to variations in skin type and the chemical composition of sunscreens, some students will experience skin reactions to certain brands. If schools provide sunscreen, parents should be informed of the type/brand so they can supply their own if necessary.

Management: Sunscreen can deteriorate and must be used before its expiry date. Even if the expiry date has not been exceeded, sunscreen may still be ineffective if not stored correctly.

Correct use: Staff, students, and parents should understand the limitations of sunscreen as a sun protection method. Most students will require supervision to ensure that sunscreen has been applied correctly. Schools could allow for this by, for example, building time for application into their programmes.

A further role for school health services is in the treatment of sunburn and, if necessary, referral to other agencies. Health services providers are also in an ideal position to compile sunburn related data, which can be used to assess whether current programmes are effective and to better target interventions. For example, if cases of sunburn are related to particular school or community activities, such as sports days, strategies can be modified accordingly. Where particular individuals or groups are affected more frequently, appropriate action can be taken respond to their specific needs.

Health service providers know the health effects of excessive UV exposure and often have firsthand experience in dealing with the consequences. Their expertise can be valuable in communicating the need for sun protection and appropriate strategies on an individual basis, in a classroom setting, and to the wider school community.

A Health-Promoting School addresses health promotion and sun protection by engaging students, school personnel, families, and community members in collaborative and integrated efforts to improve health in the school and through school/community projects and outreach. Healthy practices in relation to UV exposure are more likely to take place if there is consistent information and support from the family and community. If this is to occur, parents and community need to be well informed, which can be achieved if schools are willing to act as leaders through role modeling and community education programmes.

It is essential that parents understand the objectives of sun protection interventions and the underlying rationale, and that they have the knowledge and skills to allow them to reinforce the appropriate health messages at home. This increases the likelihood that parental attitudes and behaviours will be consistent with those of the school, and that parents will provide the things their children need to protect themselves, such as clothing, sunscreen, and sunglasses.

Tapping in to the concern that parents feel for their children's health is also one means of persuading them to be more proactive about their own health and that of other family members. While improving parents' sun protection behaviour may be one way of promoting sun protection for their children, the reverse may also be true: The messages children take home can encourage parents to adopt more sun protective behaviours themselves.

Although this is not an objective of school based interventions, given that, with the exception of sunburn, most of the effects of UV exposure are long term, greater parental awareness of the risks of UV exposure may also facilitate community interventions focusing on secondary prevention. If parents are aware of the signs of UV damage, they may be more likely to seek further information and early treatment, which will generally improve health outcomes.

Sun protection interventions can be a means of involving the broader community in school based activities. Health services can deliver health education programmes that provide knowledge about the consequences of UV exposure and how to reduce the risk of damage, or provide advice about content and presentation. Resources can be developed jointly and shared between the school and the community.

Community members who have themselves experienced health problems relating to UV exposure are often willing to provide firsthand accounts to others. The value of this type of participation is enhanced if those providing the information are respected by students, for example, successful sports people. In return, these people often appreciate the opportunity to "give something back" by encouraging young people to take preventive measures. Cooperation with local businesses can guarantee the availability and promotion of sun protection items.

Any promotion of sun protection strategies within the community will serve to further spread and reinforce the message beyond those with direct links to the school. In turn, the school can demonstrate leadership by incorporating sun protection interventions into all of its activities and thus acting as a role model for the community. Sports days and school fairs are all ideal opportunities for the school to showcase its sun protection strategies.

The media, including television, radio, signboards, posters, calendars, newspapers, magazines, and leaflets, can be used to raise awareness and to encourage more sensible sun exposure. This can occur on any scale, from local to national, and is an effective means of communicating simple messages that can be further developed through more comprehensive education programmes. Securing the cooperation of media that appeal particularly to young people can help to ensure that messages consistent with sensible sun behaviour are promoted.

For example, information on the ageing effects of sun exposure can be included in articles on skin care in magazines targeting young girls. Recruitment of successful sports people or celebrities with whom students can identify through the media is one way to influence young people's behaviour. If such people are seen to behave sensibly in relation to sun exposure and protection, there is a greater likelihood that young people will do the same.

While schools themselves seldom have the resources to secure the services of such people, developing partnerships with other agencies that do-for example, government and nongovernmental organizations, business, and national sporting bodies can-is one way of gaining access to them. Techniques used in the media are often subtle and pervasive; for example, use of darkly tanned models in skimpy clothing may be used to promote a range of goods intended for young people, reinforcing the view that the behaviour and appearance thus portrayed is necessary for acceptance.

Physical exercise, recreation, and sports Involvement in outdoor activities, including sports and recreation, forms an important part of a healthy lifestyle but may also increase one's risk of excessive sun exposure. However, active participation in outdoor activities need not be compromised, and, in fact, enjoyment can be enhanced through the implementation of sun protection interventions. Sensible behaviour is relatively simple to incorporate; it can also minimize risks and eliminate negative consequences, such as sunburn, that are often associated with being outdoors.

Developing appropriate sun protection attitudes and habits that can be extended from the school environment to other settings is the best means of enhancing one's good health. One way of integrating sun protection and physical exercise is through activities or games that combine the two. Examples of this are provided below. Such activities can incorporate discussions and other techniques to reinforce educational messages.

Sun protection strategies can also be incorporated in all sports and recreational activities conducted by the school, for example:

- *Developing sun protective sports uniforms or dress codes*
- *Attempting to conduct sports activities and lessons outside the peak UV periods*
- *Using shaded areas for activities where possible*

6

Infectious Disease: Challenges of School-aged Children

Health education programs offer opportunities to teach children how to avoid exposure to infectious diseases; Entry into kindergarten, as well as into seventh grade, provide important population-based safety nets to ensure that students are immunized and Reductions in communicable diseases and improved student attendance enhance the educational process. Yet as we enter the 21st century, new challenges face school-based infection control programs. They include concerns among parents about vaccine safety, confusion about immunization requirements and medical / religious exemptions, and the role of the school in responding to a bioterrorism event.

Vaccination is considered by public health experts to be 1 of the 10 greatest public health achievements of the 20th century. As a result, there has been an overall 99% reduction in the number of cases of vaccine preventable diseases reported in recent years. Also as a result, many parents, providers, and school health personnel have not witnessed the devastation caused by polio, diphtheria, pertussis, measles and congenital rubella infection.

In addition, some may not believe that varicella is a serious childhood illness, despite data to the contrary. As vaccine preventable diseases have dramatically decreased, parental concerns about vaccine safety have increased. Some parents also believe that children are getting 'too many' immunizations and that immunizations could weaken their immune systems.

A recent survey of school health personnel, including some in Massachusetts, identified similar concerns. Today much information about vaccines and their possible side effects is available through the Internet and lay press. However, this information may be anecdotal and without scientific basis. Fortunately, many published studies and expert committees reviewing available data have not yet found credible associations between vaccines and conditions such as multiple sclerosis, diabetes, autism, or other chronic diseases, nor any evidence that vaccines weaken the immune system.

Traditionally, school entry has been a time to identify children who are not fully immunized. It is also an ideal opportunity to identify students whose religious or medical exemptions may actually be due to parental concerns about immunizations. In order to respond to these concerns, school nurses and physicians must be knowledgeable about the current vaccine safety issues, as well as the latest scientific information.

In the 21st century, school heath personnel will also need to become familiar with the continually evolving information about anthrax, smallpox and other bioterrorism (BT) agents, as well as other infectious disease emergencies. They also need to become involved with their local planning committees, as schools will surely play a major role in any community-based response, including immunization efforts.

Because school nurses and other school-based health personnel have daily opportunities to talk with families, they are in a unique position to emphasize the importance of infection control techniques, immunizations, and emergency readiness. Armed with current knowledge about these issues, they can be a powerful force in promoting the health and safety of the Commonwealth's children.

In US, the federal McKinney-Vento Homeless Assistance Act, reauthorized in January 2002, ensures educational rights and protections for children and youth experiencing homelessness. The Act clearly states that if a does not have immunizations or immunization or medical records, the Homeless Education Liaison must immediately assist in obtaining them, and the student must be enrolled and permitted to attend school in the interim. Each school district must appoint a Homeless Education Liaison.

School nurses should request that the Homeless Education Liaison obtain the student's immunization records from the school he/she last attended. The Coordinated School Health Program, a CDC collaboration between the Massachusetts Department of Public Health (MDPH) and the Massachusetts Department of Education (MDOE) to support comprehensive school health education and coordinated school health programming, offers no-cost training on the).

The Massachusetts Department of Public Health (MDPH) Abstinence Education Media Campaign has recently produced an audio CD with a facilitator's guide. This two-part, interactive discussion program was created to assist youth advisors and health educators in communicating the benefits of sexual abstinence to middle school youth, covering issues such as respectful relationships and healthy communication with adults.

The terrorist events of last fall highlight the importance of preparing for bioterrorism and other infectious disease emergencies. School health personnel may be the first to suspect an unusual health event in the community, and the first to identify an actual outbreak. Just the threat of bioterrorism can cause disruption, fear and panic.

Schools with policies and procedures in place will be best able to respond to these challenges. An infectious disease emergency is an event with one or more of the following characteristics: (a) significant public health impact, (b) infectivity and risk of transmission, (c) intervention necessary to prevent and control infection, and (d) fear and panic, sometimes widespread.

Many school health personnel have experience with infectious disease emergencies. An example is a student seriously ill with meningitis caused by Close contacts must be identified and treated, and there may be widespread concern among parents, teachers, and the media.

In a post-9/11 world, preparing for infectious disease emergencies in schools may be as simple as providing health services to students, with enhanced awareness of the potential for an infectious disease emergency and bioterrorism. Or preparation may be more complex, involving school and community planning for a range of possible emergencies. Bioterrorism is the intentional or threatened use of a biologic agent to hurt people, create fear and/or disrupt society.

Bioterrorism may or may not result in an infectious disease emergency. As we learned last year, the threat of bioterrorism, or imagined threat, is sufficient to close workplaces, initiate HazMat team responses, and create fear. During the anthrax incidents, the State Laboratory Institute tested over 3000 items for anthrax. All results were negative.

Every community in Massachusetts is required by law to have a Local Emergency Planning Committee (LEPC). These groups should include representatives from public health, emergency management, public safety, hospital and medical communities, business and civic organizations, the local school district and school health. Within schools, the comprehensive school safety plan should address a range of infectious disease emergencies.

Planning should involve public health, public safety, and emergency management personnel. The plan should address such challenges as (a) maintaining essential school services with high absenteeism (staff and students), (b) communication with staff and students after school hours, (c) communication with media, and (d) guidelines for evacuation, or "shelter in place." Plans should be reviewed, exercised and updated regularly.

As parental concerns about vaccine preventable diseases and their complications have waned, questions and misconceptions about vaccine safety have increased. Another recent survey of school health personnel, including some in Massachusetts, identified similar concerns. With that being said, the question on the minds of many parents when faced with vaccinating their children against disease is, "Are vaccines safe?" If you define "safe" as being free from any possible negative effects, then the answer is no. All vaccines do carry some degree of risk, as do all medicines. All vaccines have possible side effects.

Although most of these side effects are mild, such as pain and tenderness at the injection site, some are more severe. When considering vaccine safety, the more important question should be, "Do the benefits of getting the vaccine (avoiding the disease) outweigh the risks (side effects)?" In Massachusetts since 1996, the newer acellular pertussis vaccine has been used with fewer side effects. Some of the more severe side effects of the original pertussis vaccine included persistent inconsoluble crying, high fever and occasionally seizures.

For this reason many parents in Japan chose not to vaccinate their children against pertussis in the late 1970's and the government suspended its use in 1975. Within 3 years, the number of cases of pertussis rose from 400 to 13,000 and the number of deaths due to pertussis increased from 10 to 130. Although the side effects of the original pertussis vaccine could be relatively severe, no child ever died from the vaccine though many died from pertussis. This example from Japan demonstrates that vaccine benefit far outweighs the risk. When considering the risk of vaccines and the risk of disease, vaccines are the safer choice.

Many reports have suggested a link between vaccination and disease because of the timing involved with receipt of vaccine and disease onset. Just because one event precedes another, does not necessarily mean that the first event caused the second. Many of the studies that have made these claims have primarily looked at children who have contracted the disease and coincidentally were vaccinated.

To determine if there is a link between vaccine and diseases, you must compare incidence of disease in vaccinated versus unvaccinated populations. Parents are also worried that children may be receiving too many immunizations and that this could overwhelm their immune systems.

There is now a wealth of information confirming the fact that vaccines do not cause these diseases mainly by showing that the incidence of disease is not higher in vaccinated vs. unvaccinated children. State laws requiring proof of immunization for school entrance have played a crucial role in increasing vaccine coverage among the nation's children and protecting them from serious vaccine preventable diseases.

In fact, current school and child care immunization requirements have virtually eliminated outbreaks of vaccine preventable diseases among children in our state. The responsibility for identifying students in need of immunization to ensure that they obtain the immunizations required for school entry rests with school officials, often school nurses.

In Massachusetts, there are only two situations in

which children who are not appropriately immunized may be admitted to school - children having medical exemptions and children having religious exemptions. A medical exemption is allowed if a physician submits documentation that an immunization is medically contraindicated (e.g., for individuals who have anaphylactic reactions to vaccine constituents or are immunocompromised). This documentation may or may not include specific contraindications.

A religious exemption is allowed if a parent or guardian submits a written statement that immunization conflicts with their sincere religious beliefs. A recent survey found that many nurses in our state thought philosophical exemptions were acceptable. However, philosophical exemptions are allowed in Massachusetts, even if signed by a physician. An example of an exemption includes a written statement by parents that they refuse to vaccinate their child because immunizations are against their own personal or philosophical beliefs.

Studies have shown that states with philosophical exemptions are more at risk for outbreaks of certain vaccine preventable diseases. The law states that unimmunized children, who do not meet criteria for medical or religious exemption, "shall not be admitted to school". However, the policies for exclusion of unimmunized or partially immunized children are developed by individual schools or school districts and are enforced at the local level.

The one exception for exclusion of unimmunized or partially immunized children is in the case of homeless children, whereby they cannot be denied entry to school if they do not have their immunization records. Persons who claim exemptions from immunization for any reason are at increased risk of contracting a vaccine preventable disease compared with immunized persons.

Therefore, in situations when one or more cases of a vaccine preventable disease are present in a school, all susceptibles, including those with medical or religious exemptions, are subject to exclusion from school. These exclusion policies have been put into place in order to protect unimmunized, susceptible students, to protect others who may have had vaccine failure, and to prevent further spread of vaccine preventable disease.

Children who are unimmunized are not only at risk themselves, but pose a danger of transmission of infection to other children who cannot be effectively immunized because they are too young or because they have medical conditions that weaken their immune systems and are not adequately protected by vaccines. Due to medical advances, the number of children receiving treatment for leukaemia, receiving organ and bone marrow transplants, and taking medications or having other conditions that weaken their immune systems is growing.

In order to be protected, these vulnerable children must rely on the community to protect them from disease exposure through community-wide vaccination. Through strict enforcement of immunization regulations and evaluation of vaccination coverage among students, children in Massachusetts will continue to be protected against vaccine preventable diseases.

Vaccination is considered by the CDC to be one of the ten great public health achievements of the 20th century. Since routine use of vaccines began, the occurrence of many common diseases has decreased dramatically. In May 1980, the World Health Organization declared the world free from naturally occurring smallpox. Polio has been eliminated from most parts of the world, with only 500 cases identified worldwide last year.

Efforts are also underway to control measles, which causes approximately one million deaths worldwide every year. As illustrated in the table below, an overall decrease of over 99% was observed in the number of cases of vaccine-preventable diseases reported in the 20th century. Although improved socioeconomic conditions, better nutrition, antibiotics and other environmental factors have contributed to the decrease in disease burden, they cannot explain the dramatic and permanent drops in disease rates observed after the introduction of vaccines.

Although vaccination has successfully and dramatically reduced morbidity and mortality in the United States, routine vaccination is still very important. Vaccines should continue to be administered for a number of reasons. Primarily, history has shown that decreased vaccination rates in many countries has subsequently led to increased levels of pertussis, diphtheria, measles, polio and other vaccine-preventable diseases. To avoid a resurgence of these diseases in the United States, it is imperative that high immunization levels be sustained.

Another important reason to continue to vaccinate is to protect those around us who are unable to be vaccinated. High immunization levels will provide community-wide protection so that diseases will be less likely to spread within the community, thereby minimizing the chance that unvaccinated individuals will be exposed. This phenomenon, known as herd immunity, is only successful when high immunity levels exist.

Routine vaccination has reduced vaccine-preventable diseases to very low levels in the United States; however, continued success depends on continuing to vaccinate. Varicella, or chickenpox, has long been thought of as a relatively mild childhood disease. The illness typically presents with an itchy rash all over the body consisting of approximately 200-400 lesions and a high fever lasting 5 to 7 days.

However, the threat of complications from varicella infection is very real. These include bacterial super-infection of skin lesions, invasive group A streptococcal infections (also known as 'flesh eating bacteria'), dehydration, pneumonia, hepatitis, encephalitis, cerebellar ataxia, and death. Prior to the introduction of the vaccine in 1995, there were over 11,000 hospitalizations (approximately two-thirds of which were in children) and about 100 deaths (almost half in children) out of the 4 million varicella infections estimated to have occurred in the U.S. yearly.

Infants and susceptible individuals who are pregnant or immunocompromised are at increased risk for complications. Complications can occur in the fetus/newborn if a woman becomes infected during the first half of her pregnancy or a few days prior to and after delivery. Following infancy, the risk of death and complications increases with age. One in five adults who get chickenpox develop pneumonia that is fatal in up to 30% of the cases. Infection in school children can provide a source of exposure for susceptible family members at home causing missed work and/or school.

Studies have shown that natural history of disease does not confer life-long immunity among all people - 5% of children may develop chickenpox more than once. Minimal risks are associated with receiving the vaccine; soreness and swelling at the sight of the shot are most common. Very few experience a fever and/or mild rash and rarely, seizures or pneumonia may develop. Transmission of the vaccine-strain virus is extremely rare.

Although a limited number of vaccine recipients may develop 'breakthrough' disease at some point, it is typically much milder than wild-type varicella. While 15% of those naturally infected develop shingles, varicella vaccine recipients have a three to four fold lower incidence. Available data from on-going studies have demonstrated that immunity from vaccination lasts at least 20 years, but is believed to be lifelong.

Lastly, high vaccination rates help protect immunocompromised individuals and infants under one year of age who are unable to receive the vaccine. High immunization rates are necessary because variable use of the vaccine can cause pockets of susceptible individuals among adolescents and adults who are at increased risk of complications. Consequently, vaccination has been shown to be the safest and most effective way of achieving immunity and protection for all.

Several vaccine manufacturers have now increased production of their vaccines to meet the national vaccine demand for most of the childhood vaccines. However, there continues to be a shortage of pneumococcal conjugate vaccine (PCV7), and the Advisory Committee on Immunization Practices' (ACIP) interim guidelines remain in place.

The Massachusetts Immunization Program (MIP) has been actively promoting vaccine safety materials produced by the Vaccine Education Centre of The Children's Hospital of Philadelphia (CHOP) during immunization assessments conducted at more than 400 pediatric provider sites in 2002. The MIP, with assistance from local boards of health, plans to distribute the videos to all public libraries later this year or early in 2003.

Handwashing: Prevents New Disease

Your mom was right-wash your hands! Starting or keeping this good habit will help prevent the spread of a variety of diseases. It is important to help teach children the correct way to wash their hands, too. Thorough handwashing will help keep schoolchildren from bringing home the "disease of the week."

Good handwashing is easy to learn and do. Lather with soap and plenty of warm, running water. Rub hands with plenty of friction for at least 30 seconds. Rinse well, and don't forget to use a paper towel to shut off the contaminated faucet handle. Some important times to remember to wash your hands include:

— *after using the bathroom*

— *after changing a diaper or helping a child use the bathroom*

— *before preparing any food*

— *after handling raw meats or poultry*

— *after touching pets, especially reptiles · after handling garbage or other dirty items —after sneezing or blowing your nose. Also, remember to remind children to wash their hands:*

— *after using the bathroom*

— *after sneezing or blowing their nose*

— *after playing with kids or the toys of kids who may be sick*

— *after playing outside*

— *before eating*

— *after touching pets, especially reptiles*

Good handwashing can lower the risk of getting sick from diarrhea and colds. Frequent handwashing also removes dirt and harmful lead toxins. Encourage your children to wash their hands regularly, and set a good example. It's something you can both do together to keep your family healthy. The Massachusetts Department of Public Health has teamed up with the Massachusetts Medical Society to spread the word about handwashing.

The Massachusetts Medical Society has launched a two-year campaign to promote the health benefits of proper handwashing. The multi-faceted campaign includes public service announcements, shopping bag inserts, posters displayed in restaurants, and the creation of a life-sized costume for the campaign mascot "Soapy." Other projects under development include an informational brochure, handwashing curriculum for young children and health care workers, and story-

based coloring book, a children's song encouraging handwashing, and radio spots starring sports figures.

The July 1997 Department of Public Health Immunization Guidelines contain the most recent requirements for children to attend daycare, kindergarten, school and college, as well as the recommended immunization schedules The guidelines are based on recommendations of the Advisory Committee on Immunization Practices (ACIP), the American Academy of Pediatrics (AAP), and the American Academy of Family Physicians (AAFP).

Students who were not vaccinated at the recommended time, but are in the process of completing their immunization series, may be allowed entry into schools. Because of established scientific rationale for administration of vaccines at minimal time intervals, those students following the "catch-up schedule" are not able to receive subsequent vaccines before school starts. This would then be considered a temporary medical contraindication for immunization.

The immunization schedule has been updated, as recommended by the Advisory Committee on Immunization Practices (ACIP) and the American Academy of Pediatrics (AAP). State-supplied varicella vaccine is intended for the following groups:

1) *all children 12-18 months of age, regardless of history of chickenpox;*
2) *susceptible sixth graders (e.g., those without a reliable history of chickenpox or varicella vaccination), or in the case of an ungraded classroom, those 11 years of age;*
3) *susceptible household contacts of*

immunocompromised individuals.

Persons are considered susceptible if they do not have a reliable history of varicella. A reliable past history is one of the following: 1) physician diagnosis; 2) good parental history or 3) serologic proof of immunity. Serologic testing of children before vaccination is not warranted, because most children without a clinical history of varicella are susceptible and the vaccine is well tolerated in seropositive persons. Conversely, most adults who do not have a reliable history of varicella are actually immune. Therefore, serologic testing before vaccination of adult staff is likely to be cost effective.

Modified Varicella Syndrome - Varicella, also known as vaccine-modified varicella, can occur in vaccinated people, who are incompletely protected post vaccination. This form of disease is usually mild and occurs 6 weeks after vaccination. Nevertheless it is transmissible to some degree, and cases should be excluded from school according to the same guidelines as unvaccinated cases of wild type disease.

Vaccine Associated Rash - Vaccine associated rash occurs in 1-5% of vaccinated persons. While it can appear within 6 weeks post-vaccination, it is most common 1-3 weeks after vaccination. Post-vaccination rash can be localized at the site of injection or generalized. In addition, persons with vaccine associated rashes are afebrile, have fewer vesicular lesions, and have shorter duration of illness than unvaccinated persons. Those with post vaccination rash are much less infectious than those with wild-type disease.

When transmission does occur it tends to result in

asymptomatic seroconversion or very mild disease in contacts, because of the attenuated vaccine strain of virus involved. While there are no official guidelines, many experts feel it is acceptable for children with post vaccination rash to attend school, provided they are otherwise asymptomatic.

School health programs will need to develop their own policies around this issue, and nurses will need to carefully evaluate the timing of the rash, the number of lesions and the general health of the child. A rash is more likely to be due to vaccine when: 1) it occurs within 1-3 weeks post vaccination; 2) has < 20 lesions; and 3) the child is afebrile and otherwise asymptomatic. A rash with these characteristics is most likely to be due to vaccine, is less infectious than wild-type disease and the child could attend school, if local policy permits.

A rash is more likely to be due to wild-type disease when: 1) it occurs less than one week or greater than 6 weeks post vaccination; 2) the child has > 20 lesions; 3) the child is febrile or otherwise symptomatic. A rash with these characteristics is more likely to be due to wild-type disease. Staff and children with wild-type disease, including modified varicella syndrome, should be excluded until all lesions have dried and crusted, or until no new lesions appear, usually by the fifth day.

There are two situations in which children who are not appropriately immunized may be admitted to school: 1) a medical exemption is allowed, if a health care provider submits documentation that an immunization is medically contraindicated; and 2) a religious exemption is allowed, if a parent submits a written statement that immunizations conflict with their sincere religious beliefs.

The reporting and control of diseases identified as posing a risk to the public health is prescribed by state regulation and law. The Reportable Diseases and Isolation and Quarantine Requirements establish isolation and quarantine requirements for cases of certain diseases and their contacts in certain high risk situations, including school settings. The laws and regulations state that unimmunized children who do not meet criteria for medical or religious exemption "shall not be admitted to school."

The hard work of many school nurses is showing great results according to the summaries that have been sent in from schools implementing the sixth grade hepatitis B school- based program. Preliminary results from schools implementing the program indicate that over half of the students participate in the program, with 88%-100% of those students participating completing the three dose series.

Many school nurses have met barriers head on and succeeded in implementing a successful program for the students. Based on the 1996-1997 seventh grade immunization survey, 30% of seventh grade students in Massachusetts had already received three doses of hepatitis B vaccine. Remember, this voluntary program only began in November 1995. Hepatitis B immunization data was not received from 31% of the schools in Massachusetts.

Various reasons were cited for the lack of data, e.g. information not included on immunization record from health care providers. New updated immunization certificates are available from the Immunization Program if you want these for your school records. Based on the number of schools participating in the program, and the number of vaccine providers immunizing this cohort, we anticipate an increase in the percent of students immunized with the hepatitis B vaccine this coming year.

With the help of community resources, at least 25 communities have successfully expanded the program this year to include hepatitis B immunization of high school students. Beginning this fall, Rotary Clubs, the Massachusetts Chapter of American Academy of Pediatrics, the Massachusetts Immunization Action Partnership and the Massachusetts Immunization Program, along with the vaccine manufacturers, will team together to assist communities that wish to expand this initiative to older teens. Plans to launch this program include mailings to all school nurses.

The high school nurse gave lectures on hepatitis B as part of the health education curriculum covering issues on health effects, mode of transmission, and the importance of being immunized.

The eye is constantly exposed to many germs, dirt and other irritants, some of which can cause eye infections. The most common eye infection in the United States is called "conjunctivitis". Cases may vary from a mild redness with watery eyes to serious infections where vision is impaired or even damaged. Conjunctivitis is an inflammation of the conjunctiva, the clear mucous membrane that covers the white part of the eyeball and the inside of the eyelids.

Signs of conjunctivitis are red and irritated eyes. Anyone can get conjunctivitis since it can be highly contagious The germs causing conjunctivitis spread easily throughout a family or classroom in a matter of days. Germs travel from one person's hands, towels, or linens to the next person's. When that person touches his face or eyes, the infection can be transferred.

Hepatitis A is a highly contagious viral disease that affects the liver and can lead to varying degrees of illness. Symptoms include fever, lack of appetite, abdominal discomfort, diarrhea, dark urine and jaundice. Hepatitis A symptoms commonly last for about 3 to 4 weeks, and some people become so sick that they require hospitalization. If you or your child have any of these symptoms, see your doctor or health care provider right away.

Hepatitis A virus (HAV) is passed through the stool (feces) of an infected person. It is usually spread by person to person contact, although about 3-8% of cases since 1983 have been associated with contaminated food or water. A diagnosis of hepatitis A in a food worker can be a worrisome and disruptive event. If a person works in a restaurant or other food handling job during his or her infectious period, it is possible that contaminated food could have been served to the public.

The board of health and state department of public health may then decide to offer people eating or working at the restaurant immune globulin (IG) injections. Public health officials make their decision based upon particular circumstances, such as when the food worker was infectious, whether ready-to-eat food was handled, and the food worker's personal level of hygiene. Good hygiene is the key to stopping the spread of Hepatitis A. People who work as food handlers should be very careful about handwashing (see the article on handwashing for tips).

Meningitis is an infection of the lining of the brain

(called "meninges") or spinal cord. Meningitis symptoms, which may appear suddenly, often include high fever, severe and long-lasting headaches, stiff neck, nausea, and vomiting. If you or your child has any of these symptoms, see a doctor or health care provider right away. You may have noticed that meningitis cases have been in the news a lot this past year. This might make you think that there have been more cases during this past year than in others, but the number of cases in Massachusetts for this year and last year are about the average of what the Massachusetts Department of Public Health usually expects.

Meningitis can be caused by many different typesof bacteria (germs). Haemophilus influenzae type b used to be the most common cause of meningitis in children under 4 years old, but the use of the Hib vaccine has successfully kept that type of meningitis rare these days. Bacteria called Neisseria meningitidis can also cause meningitis. This type of bacteria is spread through close contact with saliva (spit), like kissing or sharing a water bottle. A lot of people carry these bacteria in their throats and do not get sick. Unfortunately, some people do seem to get very sick from those same germs.

When someone has meningitis from this bacteria, the Department of Public Health will ask people in close contact with the sick person to get antibiotics to protect themselves. Viruses can also cause meningitis. These viruses can be spread through sneezing and coughing. These viruses can also be shed in the feces, so people who don't wash their hands may end up with the germs on their hands. People can protect themselves and others by washing their hands often, especially after going to the bathroom, sneezing, coughing, or wiping their noses. Antibiotics are not useful to treat or prevent meningitis or other infections when they are caused by a virus.

There is a vaccine for Neisseria meningitidis, but this shot is not given as part of routine vaccinations. The number of people in this country who would get meningitis from Neisseria is too low to make the vaccine worthwhile. Plus, it does not protect the person for the rest of his/her life-only for a short time.

If a child in your son or daughter's school has meningitis, your school nurse, local board of health, and the Massachusetts Department of Public Health will all be working together to make sure that any close contacts of the sick child get the proper treatment that they need.

Preventing HIV/AIDS

In school, young people learn about sexuality, HIV, AIDS and STI in informal as well as formal ways. Therefore, we must ensure that our formal sources of learning provide accurate information that can reduce undue fear and prejudice and enable young people to protect themselves, both now and in the future. The HIV pandemic continues into the 21st century because of ignorance and our inability to help each other take better control over the circumstances that can lead to infection. Schools can help overcome both of these barriers.

WHO's Global School Health Initiative is a concerted effort by international organizations to help schools improve the health of students, staff, parents and community members. Although definitions will vary, depending on need and circumstance, a "Health-Promoting School" can be characterized as a school constantly strengthening its capacity as a healthy setting for living, learning and working. The extent to which each nation's schools become Health-Promoting Schools will play a significant role in determining whether the next generation is educated and healthy.

The term "HIV" stands for the Human Immunodeficiency Virus. This virus destroys the body's immune system so severely that it cannot fight certain diseases. While an HIV-infected person can live for many years without major health problems, the virus' destructive effects will eventually result in Acquired Immune Deficiency Syndrome, or "AIDS". People with AIDS become increasingly vulnerable to diseases and ultimately die from diseases that their immune systems and medicines cannot fight.

Research is showing that early treatment with a combination of medicines can delay the development of AIDS in people infected with HIV. Sexually Transmitted Infections, or "STI", is a general term for infectious diseases that are spread through sexual contact. HIV/AIDS can be regarded as an STI. Other major STI are syphilis, gonorrhoea and chlamydia.

Today, HIV infection is one of the major causes of disease and death among persons aged 25-44. It has already taken millions of lives and caused enormous personal, social and economic losses throughout the world. Education about HIV can help to prevent new HIV infections and reduce suffering and economic loss. Ignorance and lack of information about HIV/AIDS fuels a great deal of prejudice, causing individuals to fear contact with people who may be infected with HIV or who have AIDS.

Since health is a fundamental human right, society is obliged to help dispel biased attitudes and prejudices that affect society's overall well-being. The school is a priority setting because it offers substantial opportunities to prevent infection and discrimination:

— *Schools provide an efficient and effective way to reach large portions of the population, including young people, school personnel, families and community members.*

— *Schools can provide interventions that help reduce infections and related discrimination in a variety of ways (learning experiences, linkages to services, supportive environment).*

— *Schools reach students at influential stages in their lives when lifelong behaviours are formed.*

— *Schools provide a channel to the community to introduce HIV/AIDS prevention efforts and advocate policies that reduce discrimination.*

At present, women and adolescents are the primary groups becoming infected with HIV in Latin America and the Caribbean. In Sub-Saharan Africa, adolescent females are becoming infected in their early teens and peak infection rates occur before age 25. Even young people, neither infected by HIV nor orphaned because of AIDS, are affected by the socio-economic consequences from the epidemic in hard-hit communities and countries.

Illnesses can come and go over a period of months or even years and differ in severity. Many people with

HIV and AIDS suffer from depression because every hour of each day they must live with the knowledge that they are ill, that they will probably grow sicker and that they will die prematurely as a result of HIV infection. In late stages of AIDS, a large percentage of people experience various forms of mental illness similar to senility.

Slowly and painfully, AIDS drains their energy and enjoyment of life. This can take many years and have devastating effects on the patients, their families and friends. In addition to suffering from the consequences of a serious illness, individuals with HIV and AIDS often suffer from isolation and condemnation and are excluded from social interaction with family and friends as well as with the community.

Patients and their families often lose access to education, their jobs and sometimes health care. Ignorance plays a large part: misconceptions about HIV and sexual orientation often result in hostility and harassment. Family and friends of people with AIDS also endure the pain of isolation, fear and despair.

People with AIDS have fewer years of life expectancy, which has severe repercussions in the social and economic sectors. Economic losses from AIDS could soon exceed total foreign aid to some seriously affected countries. AIDS cripples not only the individual who suffers from the disease but their immediate communities and society at large. HIV/AIDS clearly affects the education sector and the quality of education provided, particularly in certain regions of the world, such as Africa.

Consequences of the AIDS epidemic include a probable decrease in the demand for education, coupled with absenteeism and an increase in the numbers of orphans and school drop-outs, especially among girls. A decrease in education for girls will have serious repercussions on progress made over the past decade towards providing an adequate education for girls and women.

Women play important roles as producers of food, managers of natural resources, income earners, and caretakers of household food and nutrition security. Giving women the same access to physical and human resources as men could increase agricultural productivity, just as increases in women's education and improvements in women's status over the past quarter century have contributed to more than half of the reduction in the rate of child malnutrition.

In many countries, increasing assets that women control also has a positive impact on the next generation, particularly on education and health. Despite improvements in building women's capabilities, gender gaps in entitlements-the resources that women can command through available legal means-continue to persist. Improvements have been greatest in increasing opportunities to invest in and make use of human capital, but smallest in assuring women's rights to natural and physical capital.

These disparities have serious consequences for wellbeing, not only for women themselves, but also for their families and for society. Empowering women is key to achieving food security. These briefs consider different strategies for empowering women by strengthening their asset base-natural and physical capital, human capital, social and financial capital-and by providing the legal and institutional framework to guarantee their command over resources.

Natural capital (land, water, trees, livestock, and other natural resources) and physical capital (buildings, houses, infrastructure such as roads and electricity, transportation, and various technologies) are the most tangible forms of assets. They play a major role not only in economic production, but also in providing security against difficult times. Rights to land and houses, in particular, also convey status and power within a community.

Yet these assets are unequally distributed between men and women. Even where women are primarily responsible for food production (as in many African societies), land is owned or controlled by men. Women acquire use rights through relationships to a man-usually a husband or father; maintaining those rights depends on continuing the relationship. As a result, women's productivity is often constrained because they do not have rights to make decisions, and often cannot get credit without land rights.

Just as significantly, women's dependence on men for use rights reduces their security because they can lose the right to use land if they are widowed or divorced. Thus, measures to increase women's control over land are important strategies to empower rural women. Women often have primary responsibility for domestic water uses like drinking, cooking, and washing.

Lack of access to clean, convenient water sources costs women millions of dollars and hours in time and labor to fetch water, and adds the burden of caring for those ill from polluted supplies. Responsibilities to collect water or care for the sick can also limit girls' school attendance. Domestic water supply programs often overlook women's productive uses of water for irrigation, household gardens, livestock, or other enterprises. Irrigation and other water supply programs need to make stronger efforts to include women and to ensure that they have decisionmaking rights over water.

Limited in their control over land, women may try to accumulate other assets, such as livestock, that are culturally and economically valuable, and provide needed micronutrients. Expanding women's control over livestock contributes to their empowerment and their family's welfare by increasing their incomes and access to nutritious food, as well as by increasing their skill base, confidence, and social networks. Roads, transportation, and communications infrastructure may also empower women by offering greater mobility for marketing, seeking health care, attending school, and networking.

This is especially important to women who are often tied to their homes. Infrastructure that supplies energy can reduce the time or drudgery for food processing, cooking, and cleaning, freeing women's time for other productive activities, caring for their families, or even much-needed recreation. Technology designed specifically to address their needs can empower women by increasing their productivity or reducing their workloads.

In contrast to natural and physical capital, there have been dramatic improvements in women's human capital capabilities in the last few decades. In the last twenty-five years, life expectancy has increased 20 percent faster for females than for males, fertility rates have declined, and gaps in educational attainment have begun to close. Such investment in women's human capital is important, since women are both agents of and beneficiaries of development.

Investment in their human capital, more than any other form of investment, increases women's capabilities, expands opportunities available to them, and empowers them to exercise their choices. And there is evidence that women, their families, and their countries-and the world, by extension-will benefit in terms of improved food and nutrition security. Improving women's education is probably the single most important policy instrument to increase agricultural productivity and reduce poverty.

Women's education also leads to lower fertility and child mortality, as well as better health, nutrition, and educational outcomes for children. Despite this, in many poor countries, notably in Sub-Saharan Africa, women's educational levels are still low, and in other regions, such as South Asia, gender gaps in schooling are still large. Policymakers have thus attempted to experiment with subsidies and service delivery schemes in order to increase women's education.

For many poor women, working as agricultural wage laborers may be their only contribution to family income. Often, women face barriers to working outside the home, resulting from cultural preferences for female seclusion, or domestic responsibilities such as childcare and providing fuel and water. Returns to female labor increase with female education, so higher rates of female labor force participation are typically observed in countries and regions with higher levels of female education. The Latin American experience suggests that progress is possible for women in the labor market, although barriers to female employment -lack of child care and racial and ethnic discrimination, for example-still exist.

Women's health and nutrition demonstrate most vividly the intergenerational payoffs to investing in women's human capital. Unlike disease, nutritional status is cumulative over time, and influences the nutritional status of the next generation. Malnutrition that occurs during childhood, adolescence, and pregnancy has an additive negative impact on the birth weight of future babies.

Social, economic, and cultural factors, as well as the biological requirements of childbirth and lactation, have led to women's higher vulnerability to malnutrition relative to men. Women need to be empowered to look after their own nutrition as well as those of their families. Working through groups is one major mechanism through which outside programs and women themselves can improve the status of women.

In fact, the networks and collective action that groups generate are being recognized as assets in themselves. Social capital may be one asset in which gender inequalities are not as pronounced, or in which women even hold an advantage. Microfinance is perhaps the best-known type of program that works through women's groups.

Group savings, credit, and insurance programs for women substitute collective action through the groups for conventional assets (such as land) as collateral. Although microfinance programs may include insurance provisions, broader safety nets are required to reduce women's vulnerability to unexpected changes in weather, prices, economy, health, or relationships.

Family and friendship networks have historically

provided some measure of social security, but they have often been inadequate for the very poor, and pressures of migration and broader change are breaking down the institutions that provided such security. Thus formal, externally assisted safety net programs with explicit provisions for women are also required. Legal and institutional frameworks provide the basis for women to legitimately lay claim to all the types of assets mentioned above.

Legal rights and voice in the political system are "political capital" that enables women to strengthen their rights over other assets. In many countries, constitutions state equality before the law as a foundation of the legal system. International conventions such as the Convention on the Elimination of Discrimination Against Women (CEDAW), the Fourth World Conference on Women in Beijing in 1995, and the follow-up Special Session of the General Assembly (Beijiing+5) have also played an important role in promoting women's legal rights and helping nongovernmental and advocacy groups in countries to make their national governments accountable.

While many countries have promulgated statutory laws to reform discriminatory customary practices, they have often had unintended effects. If women are poor and uneducated, they may not be aware of the provisions of the law. Egalitarian laws and norms work best when both men and women have economic opportunities. Reforming the legal system and increasing women's asset base are thus complementary activities needed for women's empowerment.

Empowering women by strengthening their control over a range of assets is critical for enhancing their welfare as well as improving the status of future generations. Gender disparities in natural and physical capital persist partly because the legal framework supports property rights systems that are biased against women. Social and cultural institutions also need to be changed to create an environment where women can realize their full potential.

Design and implement creative programs enabling women to use and benefit from their own resources and capabilities. Such programs could include groups that provide women opportunities to build social capital or substitute for their lack of physical and financial assets. Increase women's ability to actively participate in the development process by changing perceptions and increasing awareness of both men and women themselves.

Women need to be empowered to make their own choices and to respond to increasing opportunities. Investing in women's human capital through education and training and removing barriers to the productive use of women's time and energy are key to sustainable and gender-sensitive food policy. Land assets, including soils, home sites, and crop, grazing, and forestland, are important everywhere.

But in countries where agriculture dominates, ownership of land is politically significant and directly associated with power. Command over property is, arguably, the most severe form of inequality between men and women today. Despite its prevalence, gender differences in rights to land are one of the most poorly documented dimensions of gender inequality and figure in few statistical systems. Poverty is inversely correlated with household land ownership. The landless are more vulnerable, especially in famines, and have higher infant mortality rates.

Women and children suffer disproportionately from shocks when their rights to household resources, including land, are mediated through men. Direct access to land minimizes women's risks of impoverishment and improves the physical well-being and prospects for her children. Even small plots provide access to natural resources that contribute to survival, security, and economic status. Furthermore, since many types of development specialists seek out only heads of household with secure tenure status, direct access to land also indirectly facilitates access to agricultural support services.

Land rights increase women's power in social, economic, and political relationships. Rural women claim that secure land rights increase their social and political status, and improve their sense of self-esteem, confidence, security, and dignity. By diminishing the threat of eviction or economic destitution, direct and secure rights to land can increase women's bargaining power in their families and participation in public dialogue and local political institutions. An important policy issue is whether customary tenure systems that are locally enforceable and have adapted over time or formal statutory systems that are legally or morally bound by universal conventions can provide women with greater and more secure access to land.

Land rights, in both statutory and customary tenure systems, fall along a spectrum that roughly corresponds to degrees of power. This spectrum accommodates diverse and fluctuating interests and provides different people with different bundles of rights. The entitlements a woman holds determine where she fits on the spectrum, from full ownership with all entitlements at one end to landlessness without entitlements at the other.

In both systems, most women are located somewhere between these two extremes. Both customary and formal tenure systems evolve and can accommodate short- term changes and opportunities. Customary systems usually regulate access to resources according to membership in a lineage, community, or household. These systems operate most effectively when land is relatively abundant and most land users know one another and have regular and direct contact.

Formal systems are most effective where land values are high and land transactions among strangers are frequent, requiring transparency and public records to reduce information asymmetries. Even in formal tenure systems, unwritten rights often coexist with the limited number of rights that are actually recorded in registries or titles. In practice, however, the codification of customary rights has often strengthened and concentrated land rights of individual, senior, male household heads over multiple other interests, resulting in only a small percentage of the population, and strikingly few women, holding land certificates or titles in developing countries.

There are essentially two ways to enhance women's land rights. One is to protect or increase the security of existing rights. The other is to create new rights or increase the range of rights over which women have control. The comparative advantage of customary tenure systems is an institutional capacity to support existing land rights, while for formal systems it is the capacity to create new rights. A woman's rights are secure when she can use or manage land in a predictable fashion for a defined length of time.

Security of tenure consists of three dimensions: definition, independent control, and enforcement. The first component is clarity in duration and content of rights. Very limited rights, such as fuel wood collection, can be secure if they endure over time. The content of customary rights can be ambiguous, however, since they are established through oral contracts that are frequently modified and reinterpreted.

A promising area for policy development is the clarification and registration of women's customary use rights. Tenure security for women could be improved by establishing contracts protecting widows and children from eviction or by developing leasehold contracts documenting the duration and scope of women's land rights to permit planning and managing of land and income use. A second component of security is independent control-a factor greatly diminished because of the derivative character of women's rights to land.

For most women, land rights are derived from their relationships to men: fathers, husbands, or brothers. The difficulty in distinguishing rights of different household members also contributes to the, sometimes false, assumption that women in landed households share these rights and that women's specific land rights need only be defined when they head households. But in most cases, unlike men, women cannot liquidate, trade, or retain derived land rights when the male link is lost.

Continued access to land depends on a woman's fulfilling or negotiating a constantly changing set of obligations and expectations defined by the men who hold the rights. A third dimension of security of tenure concerns women's ability to defend and enforce their land rights. Tenure security depends upon women's capacity to lobby for and promote their interests and upon whether the formal and customary authorities vested with the power to protect women's land rights share these interests and have a strong imperative to uphold them.

For improvements in tenure security to become operational, they need to be socially acceptable to formal and informal governing bodies with different norms and values. Policymakers need to identify partners capable of influencing the attitudes, priorities, and incentives that govern political and group decisions. Proposals for improved tenure security also need to be administratively viable.

Customary land institutions are familiar and convenient to rural women, reducing the transaction costs that prohibit recourse to formal land administration services. But this social and physical proximity can also be repressive. Government offices and land registries can introduce new principles, maintain public land records, and offer a neutral forum in which women can effectively press their claims, but require transparent and consistent procedures and affordable transaction costs.

In many countries, these institutions are inefficient, corrupt, time consuming, and complex. Few women have the political connections, know-how, money, or physical proximity needed to secure land rights within them. A challenge for government planners is to build a land administration capacity capable of more efficient land transfers than customary inheritance systems. Another challenge is to develop a robust, affordable and accessible dispute resolution procedure.

Such a procedure needs to have a quasi-judicial footing, consistency in its operation, impartial and informed officials, a court-based appeal process, and the support of both men and women. Where there is political will, formal tenure systems can be better suited than customary ones to rapidly creating new land rights for women. However, two major formal mechanisms-land reform and land markets-have not resulted in positive change.

Land reforms associated with new political regimes and government-or project- based land redistribution have induced significant changes in landholding patterns, poverty, and inequality while adversely affecting women almost universally. Only an estimated 4 to 25 percent of the beneficiaries of Latin American land reforms in the 1960s and 1970s were women. Similarly low percentages continue to characterize donor-driven resettlement and irrigation projects.

Clearly, to improve women's property rights, land reform policy must focus political will on favoring women in redistribution through stable, capable institutions. Changing policies that regulate land markets is a second formal mechanism for creating new rights. However, where women can legally purchase land, in practice only wealthier women and women's groups have the income to compete in the market.

Nepotism, preferential treatment, and complex, expensive procedural requirements restrict entry to land markets. Policy should focus on reducing the administrative transaction costs and barriers faced by poorer buyers and women. Women do not form a single group or always act in solidarity. Coalition building and negotiated reform can help to induce positive change.

Cross-sectoral alliances, unions, and lobby groups can build a shared awareness of common positions among women, encouraging joint action. Women and like-minded citizens who have formed viable civil society groups or cooperatives have, on a small scale, not only succeeded in purchasing land, but have also increased their capacity to leverage relationships of power and manipulate public opinion and legal contexts. These shifts in public attitudes are critical for creating the convergence of values that support changes in tenure systems.

Complementary policies must address women's limitations in exercising and enjoying their land rights. Even with assured land rights, investments in property require access to financial markets and information, extension, and other services. Policymakers should be aware of the complexity of tenure systems and how legal principles associated with land rights can be subverted when put into practice.

Water used for drinking, cooking, washing, and cleaning contributes to the welfare of all household members. Like other responsibilities for household welfare, the responsibility to provide water for consumption is gendered. In rural communities men may be responsible for the construction and maintenance of domestic water infrastructure, while women ensure that water is permanently available in the home, although other patterns have been reported as well. When the government or private vendors sell domestic water for cash, either men or women or both *may be responsible for that household expenditure.*

The gender issue at stake is the intrahousehold division of responsibilities for household welfare. A common long-term vision is that spouses should equally share these unpaid domestic chores. In the short run, however, in poor urban and rural areas, the main issue is that poor men, but especially poor women, need to be liberated from the often exorbitantly high cash or labor costs for mediocre water service and low-quality sanitation.

What is widely recognized as a basic human right, namely access to safe drinking water and sanitation, needs to be concretized. Whether the private sector or public sector is most effective in realizing this right is an open issue, but public financial support remains necessary.

In any case, water supply projects become considerably more effective if men's and women's complementary intrahousehold roles and perspectives are incorporated in project design and implementation, up to decisionmaking levels. Water as input in farming and other productive activities generates an income that is mainly controlled by the manager of the enterprise.

Young people are society's greatest asset and deserve strong investments from society. Supporting schools is one way to invest in youth and prepare them to lead satisfying and productive lives. Investments in youth can benefit nations and communities, as well as individuals. However, such investments cannot yield their full benefit if HIV/AIDS, STI, sexual violence, unintended pregnancy and other preventable health problems disrupt the learning and lives of students.

Effective HIV/STI intervention is needed to maximize investments in youth and bring about intended improvements in equity, social and economic development and productivity. By responding strongly to the challenge of HIV/AIDS, the education sector can help reduce the future impact of this disease on overall development.

Schools need to educate community members and work with them to determine the most appropriate and effective ways to prevent HIV infection among young people HIV prevention requires discussion and consideration of taboo and complex issues, such as sexuality, substance use and related beliefs that are rooted in religion, culture and law. Some parents and community leaders regard education about sexuality and related issues as family or religious matters and not as appropriate topics for school.

Yet, parents often lack factual information and/or have difficulty addressing these issues with adults as well as with children. Some parents rely on schools to educate their children in ways they themselves cannot. Opinions and needs vary from school to school and from community to community. It is clear however that in any community schools alone cannot decide the most appropriate way to help young people learn about HIV prevention. Community members must be well informed and closely involved in making such decisions.

Schools need to educate their community members and create forums for debate and discussion so that, together, they make decisions that can equip young people with the knowledge and skills needed to prevent

HIV/STI and related discrimination.

Policies and curricula can provide highly visible opportunities to demonstrate a commitment to equity, gender and human rights Schools, traditionally, are the institutions that model society. Within the context of this "model" society, students learn skills needed to make decisions about complex issues. Schools promote objectivity, inquiry and debate as a part of the learning process, and by their very nature can further discussion of social issues such as equity, gender and human rights.

HIV/AIDS challenges equity, gender and human rights. The school can either be a place that practices discrimination, prejudice and undue fear, or it can be a place that demonstrates, in a highly visible manner, society's commitment to:

Equity

Schools can ensure that "every child and every adolescent has the right to education", especially education that is necessary for survival. According to the Convention on the Rights of the Child, the right of children, even those with impairments, to receive education should not be circumvented under any circumstances. In response to the challenge of HIV, young people need to receive information about HIV/AIDS/STI and the risk of HIV/STI. Pupils infected with HIV should have the same educational opportunities as others.

Schools can ensure that both girls and boys receive complete information about HIV/STI and their prevention, and that both young men and women are taught about risk behaviour, respect and care for partners.

Gender Specificity

Worldwide, rates of HIV infection are increasing among women. Women are physically more vulnerable to HIV infection than men. They are also socially and economically more vulnerable to conditions that force people to accept the risk of HIV infection in order to survive. In Africa, south of the Sahara, there are already six women with HIV for every five men with HIV. Yet in many places, schools are apprehensive about providing sex education or discussions of sexuality because of cultural demands to protect young women from sexual experience.

Thus, women often lack the skills needed to communicate their concerns with their sexual partners or to practice behaviours that reduce their risk of infection. In addition, women are often subject to systematic interpersonal and institutional inequalities; important methods of HIV/STI prevention, such as condoms, are controlled by men. Gender-specific education can help women address such structural and interpersonal inequalities.

Human Rights

Schools can provide knowledge and help people to acquire skills that are needed to avoid HIV/STI and related discrimination. Those who are economically, socially or legally deprived have little or no access to HIV/STI prevention programmes. The school may be the only channel for reaching the deprived (especially women) with knowledge and skills for their well-being.

Professional educators, regardless of moral or political convictions, are bound to protect and promote the human and civil rights of all people and help people recognize the psychosocial damage caused when human rights are denied, whether for reasons of religion, culture, gender or sexual orientation.

The specific behaviours which spread HIV infection are well defined. Schools have been successful in teaching young people that HIV is spread from an infected to an uninfected person through: unprotected sexual intercourse; shared use of unsterilized drug injecting equipment, and skin piercing, tattooing and shaving equipment; blood transfusions (though only in countries where blood screening is not routine); and from an infected mother to her child during birth or breast-feeding.

Schools can help prevent and reduce the risk of HIV infection among young people Schools have been successful in helping young people acquire the knowledge, attitudes and skills needed to avoid infection. Education, when it is appropriately planned and implemented, is one of the most viable and effective means available for stopping the spread of HIV infection.

Evaluation studies of HIV/AIDS education have identified the characteristics of school programmes that are effective in persuading students to adopt safer sexual practices. Effective programmes focus on specific risk-taking behaviour, are based on social learning theory, use active and personalized teaching methods, provide instruction on how to respond to social pressures, reinforce social norms against unprotected sex, and offer opportunities to practice communication and negotiation skills. Also, programmes that promote postponement of sex and protected sex have been found to be more successful than programmes that promote abstinence alone.

HIV prevention interventions can have a broad impact on students' health and the classroom environment HIV/AIDS/STI interventions in schools can teach behaviours that will empower children to make healthy choices related to sex and other health issues. They can provide children with opportunities to learn and practice life skills, such as decision-making and communication skills, which in turn, can help enhance other important areas of adolescent development.

HIV/AIDS interventions that deal with personal beliefs and use participatory techniques can also lead to closer bonds between the teacher and the class and demonstrate to the school population and community that the school cares for its students. Sex education will not lead to early sexual activity Researchers in many different cultural and ethnic settings have studied whether sex education leads young people to engage in sexual intercourse much earlier than they would if they had not received sex education.

A 1997 UNAIDS review of 53 studies, which assessed the effectiveness of programmes to prevent HIV infection and related health problems among young people, concluded that sex education programmes do not lead to earlier or increased sexual activity among young people. In fact, the opposite seems to be true. Twenty-seven studies reported that HIV/AIDS and sexual health education neither increased nor decreased sexual activity and attendant rates of pregnancy and STI.

HIV prevention interventions in schools can benefit the entire community as well as students In many places, schools are a vital, central component of the community; school decisions and actions directly affect many community members. Families of children in the schools may lack education themselves but hope to learn from their children. This is particularly true of migrant populations or disadvantaged socio-economic groups.

Young people, who are adequately informed, can play a positive role in helping prevent HIV/STI. They can spread their knowledge to family members and others in their communities. Through their daily interactions, school/community projects, drama or print media, they can reach out to the community and foster discussion and debate, reflection and learning.

The first step in efforts to prevent HIV/AIDS/STI and related discrimination is to recognize this as a priority for both health and education. The next step is to plan the interventions. This will involve determining which strategies will have the most significant influence on health, education and development and how to integrate interventions with other health promotion efforts for maximum results. Following are the key steps to consider in planning HIV/AIDS/STI interventions as an essential element of a Health-Promoting School:

— *Establishing a School Health Team and a Community*

Advisory Committee

— *Conducting a situation analysis*

— *Fostering political and cultural acceptability*

— *Developing school policies, intervention goals and objectives*

Health-Promoting Schools involve members of the school and the community in planning programmes that respond to local needs, have community support and are likely to be maintained.

School Health Team

A School Health Team is a group of people working together to maintain and promote the health of all people who are working and learning at school. Ideally, the team coordinates and monitors health promotion policies and activities, including those related to HIV/AIDS. Potential members include: teachers, administrators, students, parents and school-based service providers, such as members of the health services. The team should include a balance of students and adults with various responsibilities in the school who are committed to the idea of health and HIV/STI prevention.

The School Health Team, or selected members, can be responsible for planning, designing and evaluating efforts to prevent and reduce HIV/STI. For example:

— *Young people, involved in an early stage of planning, can help develop a programme that responds to their specific needs and concerns.*

— *Parents and teachers can help ensure that*

programmes are developed in a culturally appropriate manner.

— *Teachers and other school staff can help ensure that interventions are developed with consideration of what they know and what they can do to establish HIV/STI prevention as an essential element of a Health-Promoting School.*

If a school does not have a School Health Team or group organized to promote health, the HIV/STI prevention effort can provide the opportunity to form one.

A Community Advisory Committee

A Community Advisory Committee can represent a wide spectrum of local groups and organizations. It can provide information, arrange resources, give advice and provide support for HIV/STI prevention. The Community Advisory Committee should include men and women with a diversity of skills who:

— *can influence students' knowledge, attitudes and behaviours related to HIV/STI prevention*

— *are influential in the community or district*

— *are interested in health promotion and HIV/STI prevention o are able to mobilize support and connections*

— *represent the community's geographical areas as well as economic, social, ethnic and religious make-up.*

It will be beneficial to include representatives of existing community groups, such as a healthy city council or local AIDS prevention committee. To facilitate the efforts of the School Health Team, the Community Advisory Committee can help to:

- *determine local needs and resources*
- *disseminate information about health and HIV/STI prevention*
- *build community support*
- *encourage community involvement*
- *help obtain resources and funding for health and HIV/STI prevention interventions*
- *reinforce learning experiences provided in school.*

The Community Advisory Committee and the School Health Team should work together to plan health promotion efforts and coordinate the various components of a Health-Promoting School, such as health education, health services and community and family involvement, so that all aspects of health promotion work together for health and HIV/STI prevention. If the school does not have a Community Advisory Committee, the HIV/STI prevention effort provides an opportunity to form one.

Policy-makers, decision-makers and interested groups at national, district and local levels should consider a situation analysis to guide the development of Health-Promoting Schools and HIV/STI prevention programmes.

A situation analysis will help people better understand the needs, resources and conditions that are relevant to planning interventions. A good situation analysis has several benefits:

- *Policy-makers and decision-makers need strong arguments, especially when their actions involve allocating resources.*

— *Accurate and up-to-date information can provide a basis for discussion, justification for action, setting priorities and identifying groups in special need for interventions, such as children living in geographical areas where HIV/STI and substance use are prevalent.*

— *Data obtained through the situation analysis can help ensure that interventions are tailored to the specific needs, experience, motivation and strengths of students, staff, families and community members. Data also provide a baseline against which to measure trends in HIV infection and related behaviours, such as condom use or shared needle use.*

The success of efforts to implement Health-Promoting Schools and education to prevent HIV/STI depends on the will, commitment, support and action of health and education authorities. Endorsement and support from leaders and senior officials are essential. Political leaders, at all levels, must be involved in supporting HIV/STI prevention interventions in schools.

Success also depends on the extent to which people in the community are aware of and are willing to support health promotion efforts. From an early stage, schools need to inform parents and community members about the design, content, delivery and assessment of the programme. Schools can then respond to their concerns and get their commitment. Community group meetings, parent-teacher associations, formal presentations, open houses, civic clubs and religious centres are useful for promoting and encouraging community involvement.

Partnerships with representatives from sectors such as education, health, business, communication, recreation, voluntary service, nongovernmental organizations and religious groups can demonstrate commitment and provide resources and support for health promotion and HIV/STI prevention. Communities can show their commitment by:

— *Public acknowledgement by local health, education, social and religious leaders of the importance of HIV/STI prevention, especially in schools. o Allocating local resources, such as public money for HIV/STI prevention interventions in schools.*

— *Coordinating school interventions and community programmes, such as HIV/STI prevention programmes, substance use prevention programmes, local testing/counselling and hospice services.*

— *Ongoing efforts to attract community attention to the problem, through HIV- and STI-related peer education, dramas, print material, community fora and mass media.*

— *Highly visible expressions of support from existing councils, school boards and organizations, such as women's groups, youth groups and civic groups.*

Goals and objectives of HIV/STI prevention interventions in schools

Goals should describe in broad terms what the programme will achieve. In a Health-Promoting School, the overall goal of HIV/STI-related interventions is to prevent HIV/STI and reduce HIV-related discrimination. A goal must be broken down into specific objectives so that everyone clearly understands what needs to be done to achieve the goal.

Objectives are steps for achieving the overall goal. Objectives may focus on health status, behaviour and/or conditions, as well as measurable changes in knowledge, attitudes, skills and services. The following list provides examples of objectives that could be developed for HIV/STI prevention interventions in middle and/or secondary schools:

— By, the percentage of students who report that they engage in sexual intercourse without a condom will be reduced from ... percent to at least ... percent as evidenced by self reported information collected in anonymous surveys of secondary school students.

— By, the percentage of students that are able to identify at least four ways that HIV is transmitted will increase from ... percent to at least ... percent as evidenced by pre- and post-test results among middle school students.

— By, the percentage of students that participate in at least one school/community project to prevent HIV/STI and related discrimination will increase from ... percent to at least ... percent as evidenced by student activity reports.

— By, the percentage of students who report that they are confident they can assert their decision not to engage in sexual intercourse with pressuring partners will increase from ... percent to at least ... percent, as evidenced by pre-post tests of middle school students.

Components of School Health Programme

A Health-Promoting School strives to use the school's full organizational capacity to improve the health of students, school personnel, families and community members. Such a school offers many opportunities to promote HIV/STI prevention. HIV/STI prevention interventions can serve as an entry point for developing or enhancing policies, planning groups and various components that serve as a framework for a Health-Promoting School. These components include, but are not limited to:

— *School health education*

— *Healthy school environment*

— *School health services / counselling and social support*

— *School / community projects and outreach*

— *Health promotion for school staff*

The effectiveness of interventions integrated into each of these components depends on how they are supported by people, policies and trained staff. Not every school will have the resources to integrate HIV/STI prevention interventions into all of the components at one time. Each school has to establish its own priorities.

A Health-Promoting School enables all parties concerned -students, parents, teachers and community members -to work together to set such priorities. It is important to start as soon as possible with small changes instead of waiting until resources become available to address all of the components simultaneously.

Overall, school health education seeks to help

individuals adopt behaviours and create conditions that are conducive to health. Thus, the clear and precise delineation of behaviours and conditions that are to be influenced is essential for the development of effective school health education efforts. Examples of behaviours commonly addressed to prevent HIV/STI and related health problems are listed below.

To help schools develop health education interventions to address such behaviours and conditions, WHO and UNESCO have developed School Health Education to Prevent AIDS and STD, a resource package containing a Handbook for Curriculum Planners, Student Activities and a Teacher's Guide.

In a Health-Promoting School, health education to prevent HIV/STI is designed to help students acquire the knowledge, attitudes, beliefs, skills and support to make informed decisions, practice healthy behaviours and create conditions conducive to health. The design must consider the developmental level of the students, starting at primary levels and continuing to secondary levels, to build on and reinforce previous learning experiences.

Important knowledge, attitudes, values and skills related to the prevention of HIV and related discrimination are described in the boxes below. Items are categorized for different developmental levels - young children, pre-adolescents and adolescents. Close collaboration between education and health officials, as well as with parents, students and community members, is necessary to determine the most important and appropriate content to provide to help young people avoid HIV and STI.

Students will learn that:

— *HIV is a virus some people have acquired*

— *HIV is difficult to contract and cannot be transmitted by casual contact, such as shaking hands, hugging or even eating with the same utensils*

— *people can be HIV-infected for years without showing symptoms of this infection*

— *many people are working diligently to find a cure for AIDS and to stop people from contracting HIV infection*

Students will demonstrate:

— *acceptance, not fear, of people with HIV and AIDS*

— *respect for themselves*

— *respect between adolescent males and females - tolerance of differences in attitude, values and beliefs*

— *understanding of gender roles and sexual differences*

— *belief in a positive future*

— *empathy with others*

— *understanding of duty with regards to self and others*

— *willingness to explore attitudes, values and beliefs*

— *recognition of behaviour that is deemed appropriate within the context of social and cultural norms*

— *support for equity, human rights and honesty*

Students and others will be able to:

— *acquire practical and positive methods for dealing with emotions and stress*

— *develop fundamental skills for healthy interpersonal communication.*

Virtually every school will have students who have in the past or who are at present engaging in risky sexual behaviour, whether by their own choice or forced by others. Students must be taught specific ways to reduce the risk of HIV/STI. Education to prevent HIV/STI and related discrimination should be an important part of a school health curriculum, integrated into various subject areas and included in the school's extracurricular activities.

School health education should be a planned, sequential course of instruction from the primary through the secondary levels, addressing the physical, mental, emotional and social dimensions of health. It can be taught as a specific subject, as part of other subjects or as a combination of both.

Education to prevent HIV/STI and related discrimination should be combined with education about life skills, reproductive health and alcohol/ substance use so that the learning experiences will complement and reinforce each other. To link these issues, organize them into a school health education curriculum and/or coordinate the simultaneous or sequential presentations of related topics in different classes.

Scientific terms and biological-technical details may seem important; however, for the purposes of health education, they are less important than practical and basic information that will enable students to avoid infection. It is more important for a student to learn how the virus is spread and how to negotiate safe sex, for example, than to learn about the composition of the virus.

Students need to also learn about the fears that surround HIV/AIDS/STI. Some students may fear risk when abstaining from sexual intercourse or engaging in common sexual activities such as masturbation. Some students may experience fear when engaging in expressions of affection such as hugging, kissing and touching genitals. Some students may fear being near or touching someone who may have acquired HIV infection.

Because of misconceptions about how HIV is and is not transmitted, some students may suffer undue anxiety and concern. Students must be taught how the virus is and is not spread. When they overcome fear, their understanding and empathy toward people who have HIV/AIDS can grow. Such information will enhance understanding among teachers, other school personnel and health workers, and will help them focus interventions on the factors that contribute most to HIV infection in the community.

This information is also important in developing complementary educational efforts such as those carried out by mass media, health workers, religious groups and other organizations. The influence of mass media is important to consider. Young people are frequently exposed to and influenced by the media. While schools teach one set of messages, the media may be providing quite different messages.

School-based programmes should take into account information provided through the mass media and take steps to refute unhealthy messages. Two essential actions are needed to tailor HIV/STI education to the specific needs of students and others in the community:

- *Identify specific behaviours and conditions most relevant to HIV/STI prevention in the community.*
- *Specifically delineate the knowledge, attitudes, belief, values, skills and services that positively or negatively influence behaviours and conditions most relevant to HIV/STI.*

Educational methods such as lectures, discussion, role-plays and audio-visual aids should be designed to influence specific factors -such as knowledge, attitudes and values, myths, skills and services -related to behaviours and conditions most relevant to HIV/STI in the community. Select an education method on the basis of how well it will influence a particular factor. For example, a lecture is an effective way to increase knowledge, but less effective in influencing beliefs and building skills. Educational methods also need to correspond with the developmental level of students and be sensitive to the cultural context.

Education about HIV/STI prevention and sexual behaviour poses a major dilemma for many educators, a dilemma fuelled by public pressures and the different beliefs and values of government, various religions and parents. As schools try to determine the most appropriate focus for HIV/STI education, the following options may be considered and discussed with teachers, parents, students and members of the Community Advisory Committee. As a strategy to prevent HIV infection in the community, each option has its own strengths and limitations.

The options are:

— *abstinence from sexual intercourse*

— *non-penetrative sex*

— *condom use*

— *monogamy with an uninfected partner*

— *abstinence from substance use*

If schools choose to help students recognize all the options for prevention, they can teach students to select options that correspond to their own standards, lifestyle, age and personal situation. Some options will only be realistic for older students. If schools choose to promote only one option, they are likely to fail to provide a viable option for a significant proportion of students. Thus, each option should be discussed and carefully considered.

Abstinence from sexual intercourse

From a medical point of view, this practice is the safest, as it reduces the chances of infection with HIV and STI through sexual behaviour to zero and is in accordance with traditional values about young people and sexuality held in many parts of the world. In practice however, young people in many countries do have sexual relationships, or may be forced to have sex, so a significant number of them may not find the option of abstinence acceptable or realistic. Many young people, who at first intend to abstain from sex, cannot maintain that intention because of peer pressure or other personal or social factors. Programmes that promote abstinence alone have proven largely ineffective in reducing sexual activity or sexual risk taking.

Non-penetrative sex

Sexual behaviours that involve the exchange of semen, vaginal fluids or blood between partners can pass HIV from an infected to a non-infected partner. These behaviours include vaginal and anal intercourse without using a condom, taking semen or vaginal fluids into one's mouth in oral sex and any sex act that involves blood contact. Abstaining from these risky behaviours virtually eliminates the chances of contracting HIV infection but does not eliminate the chance of contracting other STI. Kissing, hugging, touching/ caressing and non-penetrative sexual activities such as masturbation do not carry the risk of HIV infection and are not likely to result in an STI. For many young people, however, and especially for adolescent males, sex means vaginal intercourse, and they may not accept the option of non-penetrative sex.

Condom use

A condom, used appropriately in connection with potentially risky sexual behaviour, considerably reduces the risk of HIV/STI. In spite of what parents and other adults tend to think, adolescents tend to be sexually active. In many countries, the average age of first sexual intercourse is about seventeen years, and in some countries the average age of initiation is even lower. Although young people usually are monogamous within a given relationship, the relationship itself lasts for a short period of time.

Most young people who are sexually active can be called serially monogamous; they do not realize that serial monogamy is identical to having multiple sexual partners. Acceptance of condom use is growing and condoms are increasingly available throughout the world. Moreover, research shows that education about condom use does not lead to increased promiscuity among young people.

Monogamy

An exclusive sexual relationship with one person can protect against HIV/STI, provided that the sexual partners are not already infected when entering the relationship and do not become infected during the relationship. However, marriage, divorce and remarriage to another partner have become increasingly commonplace in many countries. Extramarital relationships pose a threat to people who rely on monogamy to prevent HIV/STI. An overwhelming majority of people disapprove of extramarital sexual relations, but in fact, most have extrumuritul uffuirs at some point during their marriages. In polygynous societies, multiple sex partners are accepted and indicate a man's social and economic status.

Substance and needle use

Drug use influences the spread of HIV directly and indirectly. An important drug use behaviour that puts people at risk for contracting HIV infection in a direct way is needle use. The behavioural objective in this case is to stop people sharing needles or to encourage them to clean shared needles prior to use. Infection through needles is not restricted to illicit drug use and may also occur with medicinal drugs (administered by injection), with preventive care (such as vitamin injections in some cases), tattooing or piercing.

Modes of transmission vary greatly depending on the cultural context and the adequacy of health care: the content of local interventions need to reflect local culture and realities. Misuse of alcohol and substance use can increase risks indirectly by lowering people's inhibitions against engaging in unsafe sexual or drug-using behaviour.

Peer education and student involvement

Participation and empowerment are key principles of a Health-Promoting School. Youth should be involved in planning school health programmes, in carrying out the activities and evaluating them in a structured way. It is well known that young people get much of their sexual health knowledge from their peers. Young people are often sensitive to peer pressure and can exert a strong influence on one another. This influence can be negative, with young people encouraging each other to engage in risk behaviours, or channelled to have a positive influence.

Research shows that when peers deliver prevention it can enhance the effects of the intervention. Peers can contribute to HIV/STI prevention interventions in formal and informal ways. Education sessions led by peers can help to spread messages about what is safe behaviour and what is not. Young people can be effective educators: they can use language and arguments that are relevant and acceptable to their fellow students.

They are capable of presenting information and skills in an informal way and in a safe atmosphere. For these reasons, they are credible and may be able to offer applicable solutions to prevention problems among their peers. Peer educators can sometimes reach groups that professionals cannot (e.g. intravenous drug-using youth, youth in prostitution, migrant youth, gay youth and marginalized youth).

In some countries, the taboo on sexuality is very evident, and the distance between teachers and students is vast. Peer education is an investment in young people. Peer educators can serve as role models and form the basis for peer support networks. They can serve as counsellors and as opinion leaders in setting the agenda, communicating values, promoting positive social norms and life-skills training.

The work of peer educators has an impact on the peer educators themselves. It offers opportunities for students to learn to care for others and to take control of their health. It can have a positive influence on their self-esteem, skills and attitudes with regard to sexuality and health.

The role of a peer educator can extend far beyond the classroom. Peer programmes provide an excellent way to link schools to community-based organizations and offer opportunities to educate a vast number of people. Students who are trained educators in HIV/STI prevention can address school classes and community youth groups, answer telephone hotlines and staff offices where students can drop by to discuss HIV/STI-

related concerns and issues.

Peer educators are relatively low cost and typically there is an abundant pool of potential volunteers. To function effectively, however, peer educators need to be properly trained and supervised. We already known that peer educators who have only been trained to transmit knowledge run the risk of being rejected by their peers because they are perceived as "know-it-alls". They need skills in counselling, empathy, decision-making, resistance to group pressure, assertiveness and building self-esteem.

Teachers play an important role in preventive education. Pre-service and in-service training for teachers is crucial if preventive education is to be effective. Teachers and their representative organizations should be involved in every stage of planning, implementing and evaluating HIV/AIDS training. In particular, teachers need to be trained to use participatory and interactive teaching methods.

In all communities, the training of teachers should be of highest priority because, for better or worse, teachers are role models for their students and other members of their community. School personnel can be strong role models if they demonstrate their willingness to learn about HIV/STI, to show compassion and empathy towards individuals infected and affected by HIV/AIDS and respect and understanding for others regardless of gender, sexual orientation or life circumstances.

An HIV/STI training programme for teachers and other school personnel should be planned with consideration to:

— *mobilizing support inside as well as outside the school o giving financial and professional incentives o designing training, based on needs of the teachers and the school situation o establishing pre- and in-service training for teachers of all grade level o providing sufficient time for on-going training*

— *allocating personnel, time, resources and authority to a staff member who will be responsible for initiating, managing and coordinating the training*

— *developing a core group of trainers or training teams that will enable all relevant teachers and school personnel to receive training in a timely manner*

— *regularly scheduling follow-up sessions or other means by which to periodically provide updates on HIV/STI or related health problems*

— *coaching by experienced trainers for those teachers who would like to have this kind of support*

— *evaluating the impact and effectiveness of the training and revision of the training format as needed*

Training should be designed with consideration to the knowledge, attitudes, beliefs, values and skills of the teachers. In all cases it should include:

— *a rationale for implementing HIV/STI education in schools o accurate information about HIV/STI prevention o accurate information about sexual behaviour, beliefs and attitudes of young people o accurate information about alcohol and substance use in relation to HIV/STI prevention o opportunities to examine the teachers' own standards and values concerning sexuality, gender roles and substance use o explanation of a wide variety of teaching methods*

- *practice that uses various methods to impart knowledge, develop attitudes and build skills related to HIV/STI prevention and responsible sexual behaviour in a way that is inspiring and effective*
- *conflict management and negotiation skills*
- *identification and discussion of gender specific issues*
- *suggestions about ways to deal with cultural and religious traditions that may present barriers to discussions about sexuality*
- *lessons about how to promote compassion and support for appropriate guidance and care for persons infected with HIV*
- *guidance about identifying and referring students with sexual health problems to appropriate services*
- *integrating HIV/STI prevention and related topics into the existing curricula*

Curricula for HIV/STI prevention and other health-related issues may be available through governmental and nongovernmental agencies and organizations, universities or teachers' unions. Teachers and students themselves can also generate supplementary materials specific to the local situation.

Healthy school environment

The school environment plays a key role in the success of HIV/STI prevention programmes. An environment that fosters understanding, caring and empathy contributes greatly to positive values, beliefs and attitudes about HIV/STI prevention among students, teachers, staff and the community. To create an environment that supports education about HIV and STI, schools must consider policies and practices, including rules, guidance and referral to services.

Developing supportive HIV/STI-related school policies is as important as designing effective HIV/STI interventions. Supportive school policies guide the planning, implementation and evaluation of efforts to promote health and prevent HIV/STI. They incorporate the input of all relevant constituents of the school community: students, teachers, parents, staff, administrators, nurses and counsellors.

Policies should meet national and local needs and standards and be adapted to the health concerns, norms and values of ethnic and cultural groups represented at school. Examples of supportive policies and regulations:

— *Required HIV/STI training for all school personnel.*

— *Required coordination between health and education authorities at local and district levels in planning and implementing HIV/STI interventions in schools.*

— *Policies for students and school personnel that support privacy, attendance, employment and infection control.*

— *Policies that support HIV/STI prevention and other health interventions for all levels of schooling, starting in the earliest grade and continuing through the last grade.*

— *Designation of a school-level coordinator with responsibility and authority to deal with health issues and concerns.*

— *Policies about curricula content, including sensitive issues like safe sex, birth control, family planning, sexual harassment and sexual orientation. o A code of professional ethics that protects students, teachers and staff from sexual harassment and abuse.*

A Health-Promoting School promotes a caring and supportive environment for people who work and study there. Students and teachers who are infected with HIV should not fear any restrictions based solely on their HIV status. There is no acceptable reason for denying education to a student infected with HIV or denying employment to a teacher infected with HIV. Efforts to develop policy for school personnel infected with HIV should aim to ensure that employers cannot take action against an employee based solely on his or her HIV status.

Policy in terms of employment must not be influenced by HIV status. Reasonable accommodations should be made for employees who are able to perform the tasks of their position with reasonable assistance. These might include: job-related aids or services, change in work site and flexibility with rest periods and occasional absences.

Policies for HIV-infected students and school personnel may state points such as:

— *Guarantee confidentiality and privacy of HIV-infected persons.*

— *Full attendance and equitable, safe and humane treatment for students and school personnel with HIV/STI should be paramount.*

— *Each decision about educational and working environment, such as use of special aids or need to accommodate persons with HIV, must be documented.*

— *Special services can be provided to assist those with limited strength or whose illness hampers their educational and/or working performance.*

— *Policies and procedures on intervention and prevention of harassment should exist to promote an environment that fosters respect and compassion as well as social growth for all students and school personnel.*

— *HIV-related disability definitions should conform to prevailing laws, where applicable.*

— *Requirements and procedures established through collective bargaining must be respected.*

Policies help ensure the social, emotional and physical well-being of HIV-infected students and school personnel. By serving all people equitably, the school promotes understanding, respect and compassion among its students, staff and community. Universal infection-control precautions are practices that schools, like other organizations, need to follow to prevent a variety of diseases. Precautions should include policies on caring for wounds, cleaning-up blood spills and disposing of medical supplies.

While these precautions are valuable in preventing certain diseases, such as flu, chicken pox or ear infections, schools must recognize that HIV is more difficult to transmit. HIV/STI are not transmitted by casual contact, such as shaking hands, hugging or using toilet seats or eating utensils. Even kissing or deep kissing does not transmit HIV.

Universal precautions are simply policies that schools put into place as safeguards for emergency situations. To diminish fears schools should inform personnel and students about the infection-control policy and address concerns through open discussion.

A Health-Promoting School dispels fear and tension among its students, teachers and staff, and promotes values of mutual respect and acceptance. It offers a safe, trustful environment. Teachers, administrators, staff and students actively display these values inside and outside the classroom. Teachers demonstrate to students that HIV-positive individuals and people who associate with HIV-positive individuals are not to be feared.

For example, a teacher might openly hug an HIV-positive student upon his or her return to the classroom after hospitalization. Promoting activities in school, like World AIDS Campaigns and AIDS Awareness Day, are ways to support people who are infected or affected by HIV/AIDS. Such activities create understanding of HIV and its broad implications. As educators, people who are HIV infected or who have AIDS have had a great impact in correcting misunderstandings and in promoting solidarity.

In many countries, the high prevalence of HIV and STI among homosexuals and men who have sex with men increases already existing homophobia and discrimination. Promoting gender equity and understanding of different beliefs, cultures, religions and sexual orientation helps ensure that all teachers, students and staff feel accepted.

In addition to providing a social climate that promotes understanding and solidarity, a Health-

Promoting School provides a physical environment that contributes to HIV/STI prevention. Examples include offering adequate information about HIV/STI in the school library, mounting posters in the hall and instituting security regulations to ensure safe travel to and from school. The school can provide facilities for storing medication needed by students and staff. Some schools have worked with local health services to make condoms accessible to students who need them.

Many Health-Promoting Schools are striving to develop and improve school health and support services. Such services become increasingly important as the number of children and young people who are affected by AIDS-related illness, death and stigma grows. In both developed and developing countries, school health services tend to be very limited in scope and HIV-related services are not commonly provided.

Thus, the following points may be useful to persons who are trying to increase support for improved school health and support services, including services that respond to HIV/AIDS.

— In many countries young people have little or no regular access to primary health care services. In some areas, the school is the only social institution with which young people have contact.

— Despite evidence that school health services are viable and effective public health interventions, and growing evidence of their need, school health services are not well developed, if available at all, in many countries. This is unfortunate because learning and academic achievement are strongly influenced by student's physical and emotional health.

— *School health services can significantly contribute to the development of young people and should be advocated as a means of community and economic development.*

— *HIV/AIDS provides an opportunity to consider and debate the need for improved and expanded school health services.*

— *As school health services are revised and new services proposed and developed, they should be planned and implemented as an integral part of the existing school health programme and available to all students, as appropriate and relevant. Services that respond to HIV/AIDS and related health problems are likely to be most effective when integrated and co-ordinated with other school health and support services.*

A Health-Promoting School can serve as a point of support and referral for students and teachers dealing with issues associated with HIV/AIDS/STI. Not all schools provide school health services, yet where resources are available, school health services can be augmented with activities that respond to HIV/AIDS/STI-related needs and concerns. Health workers who provide school health services could make the following contributions. To help strengthen school/community response to HIV/AIDS/STI, health workers could:

— *Advocate for supportive school policies and strong school programmes with policy- and decision-makers and relevant community leaders.*

— *Engage and support education officials and representatives from other relevant sectors in providing information, building skills and providing counselling services in the school setting (and be actively involved in these efforts themselves).*

— *Collaborate with school officials, students and teachers to mobilize school and community support for efforts that respond to HIV/AIDS/STI.*

For example, develop peer networks among students that promote understanding about and support for healthy sexual attitudes and behaviours, prevention programmes and care; and link such networks to relevant programmes and networks in the school and community.

To help prevent HIV/AIDS/STI among students and school personnel, health workers could:

— *Provide information and advice to students and school personnel.*

— *Provide opportunities for school personnel, students, and parents to ask questions and clarify any doubts or concerns they may have about HIV/AIDS/STI and methods of prevention.*

— *Serve as a confidant to whom students and school personnel can express fear and anxiety about HIV/AIDS/STI without facing ridicule or judgement.*

— *Provide health products (such as contraceptives and condoms) when they are permitted to do so, by prevailing laws and policies.*

— *Identify and collaborate with organizations, which can provide appropriate non-health services when required, such as legal support for adolescents who are being abused.*

A Health-Promoting School addresses health and HIV/STI prevention by engaging students, school personnel, families and community members in collaborative and integrated efforts to improve health, both in the school and through school/community projects and outreach. Students can practice and share what they learn in the

Bibliography

Chambers, C.M., *An evaluation of the World Food Programme (WFP) / JAMAICA 2727 School Feeding Programme. Cajunas.* 24(2): 91-102, 1991.

Chandler, A.M., Walker, S.P. et al., "School breakfast improves verbal fluency in undernourished Jamaican children", *Journal of Nutrition*, 125(4): 894-900, 1995.

Chang, S.M., Walker, S.P., Himes, J. & Grantham-McGregor, S., "The effects of breakfast on classroom behaviours in rural Jamaican school children", *Food and Nutrition Bulletin*, 17: 248-257, 1996.

Del Rosso, J.M., "School feeding programs: Improving effectiveness and increasing the benefit to education", *A guide for Program Managers*, Partnership for Child Development/World Bank, 1999.

Grantham-McGregor, S., Powell, C. & Fletcher, P., "Stunting, severe malnutrition and mental development in young children", *European Journal of Clinical Nutrition*. 43: 403-409, 1989.

Hadidjaja, P., Bonang, E., Suyardi, M.A., Abidin, S.A.N., Ismid, I.S. & Margono, S.S., "The effect of intervention methods on nutritional status and cognitve function of primary school children infected with Ascaris lumbricoides", *American Journal of Tropical Medicine and Hygiene*, 59(5): 971-795, 1998.

Ivanovic, D., Vasquez, M. et al., "Nutrition and education", II. Educational achievement and nutrient intake of Chilean elementary and high school graduates, Archives of Latin American Nutrition. *41(4): 499-515, 1991.*

Jennings, J. et al., "Managing Successful Nutrition Programmes", ACC/SCN State-of-the-Art-Series, Nutrition Policy Discussion Paper No. *8, 1991.*

Leslie, J. & Jamison, D.T., "Health and nutrition considerations in education planning. 1. Educational consequences of health problems among school-age children", Food and Nutrition Bulletin. 12: 191-203, 1990.

Pollitt, E., "Malnutrition and infection in the classroom", UNESCO, Paris,1990.

Pollitt, E., Cueto, S. & Jacoby, E.R., "Fasting and cognition in well- and undernourished schoolchildren: a review of three experimental studies", American Journal of Clinical Nutrition, 67(suppl.): 779S-784S, 1998.

Popkin, B.M., Richards, M.K. & Montiero, A., "Stunting is associated with overweight children of four nations that are undergoing the Nutrition Transition", Journal of Nutrition, 126: 3009-3016, 1996.

Simeon, D.T. & Grantham-McGregor, S.M., "Nutritional deficiencies and children's behaviour and mental development", Nutrition research reviews. 3: 1-24, 1990.

World Health Organization, "Healthy Nutrition: An essential element of a Health-Promoting School", WHO/HPR/HEP/98.3, 1998.

Index